Praise for *Great Sex, Naturally*

*"**Great Sex, Naturally** is the book we've all been waiting for . . . a fabulous must-read for every woman who wants to enhance her health and sex life with natural methods. Packed with valuable and credible advice and thoroughly researched gems of information, it's written in a clear and engaging style. I wholeheartedly recommend this valuable book! Every woman should have a copy in her library."*

— **Joan Borysenko, Ph.D.**, author of *Minding the Body, Mending the Mind* and *Fried: Why You Burn Out and How to Revive*

"An essential guide for every woman—loaded with practical tips, modern naturopathic secrets, and ancient wisdom. It offers exciting tools for enhancing sexuality and health that are valuable to women of all ages. Bravo!"

— **Michael T. Murray, N.D.**, author of the *Encyclopedia of Natural Medicine*

"This wonderfully unique book is highly recommended for any woman to recharge both her well-being and her sexual vitality. It provides an abundance of libido-enhancing information that's not available anywhere else. I know that women will benefit immensely from this remarkable resource."

— **Elizabeth Lipski, Ph.D.**, author of *Digestive Wellness*

GREAT
SEX,
NATURALLY

Also by Dr. Laurie Steelsmith and Alex Steelsmith

NATURAL CHOICES FOR WOMEN'S HEALTH:
How the Secrets of Natural and Chinese Medicine Can
Create a Lifetime of Wellness (Three Rivers Press)

Hay House Titles of Related Interest

YOU CAN HEAL YOUR LIFE, the movie, starring Louise L. Hay & Friends
(available as a 1-DVD program and an expanded 2-DVD set)
Watch the trailer at: **www.LouiseHayMovie.com**

THE SHIFT, the movie, starring Dr. Wayne W. Dyer
(available as a 1-DVD program and an expanded 2-DVD set)
Watch the trailer at: **www.DyerMovie.com**

THE BODY "KNOWS": How to Tune In to Your Body and
Improve Your Health, by Caroline M. Sutherland

ECSTASY IS NECESSARY: A Practical Guide, by Barbara Carrellas

MANOPAUSE: Your Guide to Surviving His Changing Life,
by Lisa Friedman Bloch and Kathy Kirtland Silverman

MEALS THAT HEAL INFLAMMATION: Embrace Healthy Living and
Eliminate Pain, One Meal at a Time, by Julie Daniluk, R.H.N.

MORE THAN JUST SEX: Because Getting Enough
Just Isn't Enough! by Ali Campbell

WOMEN, SEX, POWER, AND PLEASURE:
Getting the Life (and Sex) You Want, by Evelyn Resh

Please visit:

Hay House USA: **www.hayhouse.com**®
Hay House Australia: **www.hayhouse.com.au**
Hay House UK: **www.hayhouse.co.uk**
Hay House South Africa: **www.hayhouse.co.za**
Hay House India: **www.hayhouse.co.in**

Every Woman's Guide to
Enhancing Her Sexuality Through
the Secrets of Natural Medicine

GREAT SEX, NATURALLY

Dr. Laurie Steelsmith and Alex Steelsmith

with Illustrations and Graphics
by Alex Steelsmith

HAY HOUSE, INC.
Carlsbad, California • New York City
London • Sydney • Johannesburg
Vancouver • Hong Kong • New Delhi

Published and distributed in the United States by: Hay House, Inc.: www
.hayhouse.com® • *Published and distributed in Australia by:* Hay House
Australia Pty. Ltd.: www.hayhouse.com.au • *Published and distributed in
the United Kingdom by:* Hay House UK, Ltd.: www.hayhouse.co.uk • *Published and distributed in the Republic of South Africa by:* Hay House SA
(Pty), Ltd.: www.hayhouse.co.za • *Distributed in Canada by:* Raincoast:
www.raincoast.com • *Published in India by:* Hay House Publishers India:
www.hayhouse.co.in

Cover design: Amy Rose Grigoriou • *Interior design:* Riann Bender
Indexer: Jay Kreider

Library of Congress Cataloging-in-Publication Data

Steelsmith, Laurie.
  Great sex, naturally : every woman's guide to enhancing her sexuality
through the secrets of natural medicine / Laurie Steelsmith and Alex
Steelsmith ; with Illustrations and graphics by Alex Steelsmith. -- 1st ed.
    p. cm.
  Includes index.
  ISBN 978-1-4019-3146-9 (pbk.)
  1. Sexual health. 2. Sex (Psychology)--Health aspects. 3. Physical
fitness. 4. Nutrition. 5. Women--Sexual behavior. 6. Self-care,
Health. I. Steelsmith, Alex. II. Title.
  RA788.S74 2012
  613.9--dc23
                        2012005727

Tradepaper ISBN: 978-1-4019-3146-9
Digital ISBN: 978-1-4019-3147-6

15 14 13 12   4 3 2 1
1st edition, July 2012

Printed in the United States of America

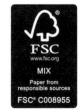

To our hanai mother,
with gratitude for her love and support

CONTENTS

PREFACE

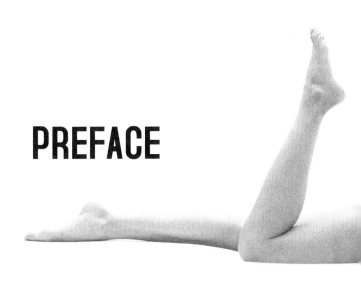

My partner and I wanted to write this book in part because thousands of my female patients have privately expressed their need to have more sexual energy, greater sexual sensation, or a deeper connection to their sexuality. And at my women's health seminars, in Honolulu and internationally during the past two decades, my presentations on sexuality and pelvic health have often been the highlight. Women seem especially eager to discover more about how they can increase their sexual energy and vitality.

We also decided to write *Great Sex, Naturally* because many books on women's sexuality focus on the mechanics of sex, but miss out on the big picture and don't address where your libido comes from in the first place. In this book, we convey a more holistic view of women's sexuality. As you read it, you'll discover many ways in which sexual pleasure can be wholesome and profoundly healing, and your sexual energy can nourish your health and transform your body, mind, and spirit. This can be greatly beneficial if you currently have a healthy sexual drive and want to further enhance it—or if you have health issues preventing you from fully experiencing your sexuality.

Many women confide in me that they have negative or anxious feelings, at the deepest level, about their sexuality. Some feel inadequate—as if they're supposed to feel something different during sex than what they actually experience. One of the goals of this book is to help women have a healthy acceptance of their feelings about their sexuality, feel more connected to their bodies, and manifest loving change in their lives.

A large part of being a healthy, vital, sexual woman is your core relationship with yourself. For a woman to have great sex, she needs to feel comfortable with, and connected to, her pelvis, her sexual organs, and the rest of her body. Many women feel disconnected from their genitals because of vaginal infections, incontinence, pelvic pain, and other conditions. A history of sexual trauma, or a cultural atmosphere that doesn't promote a positive relationship between a woman and her body and sexuality, can result in a stifled libido and diminished sexual health.

In my practice as a naturopathic physician with a specialty in women's health, I've found the natural protocols in this book highly effective for boosting women's sexuality, health, energy, and creative drive. One woman's story seems to sum up the experience of many others. She had lost interest in sex, was gaining weight, and was often exhausted. She came to see me after consulting many medical doctors, who had overlooked key signs that her body was imbalanced, said her problems were normal for her age, and recommended she simply exercise more and eat less. I found she had many symptoms and underlying imbalances preventing her from feeling amorous, including irritable bowel syndrome, vaginal dryness, and headaches. Tests revealed intolerance to gluten, high cholesterol, high blood sugar, and low sex hormones. With the right diet, bioidentical hormones, acupressure, and nutritional support, all her complaints disappeared, and her vitality and robust sex life returned.

There are countless women who similarly feel unable to make the changes they need to regain their sexual health. Many need only the right support and guidance to turn their lives around. If you're one of these women, or one of the many who simply want to enhance their sexuality, you're about to begin a journey in which you can fully manifest your potential for great health and great sex.

To your health,
Dr. Laurie Steelsmith

❖ ❖ ❖

As both Laurie's partner and a professional writer with a strong interest in natural medicine, I find it especially meaningful to co-author, as well as illustrate, this book. In its pages, you'll notice that the "voice" is occasionally in the first-person plural ("we"), and at other times in the first-person singular ("I"). Of course, "we" is Laurie and me, and "I" represents her. As in our previous book, *Natural Choices for Women's Health,* I take the liberty of writing in the first-person singular on her behalf. But although my job is to create the text, you can rest assured that I never give medical advice. (I have no formal degrees in medicine.) People often ask how we work together and exactly what my role is in writing our books, so let me take this opportunity to give you a quick sketch.

We typically talk about ideas for months, or years, before committing anything to paper. When we're ready to begin, Laurie writes down the appropriate medical information. This usually consists of the specific treatments, procedures, and protocols she recommends—the core prescriptive material, drawn from her many years of seeing patients. Much of what she writes down is in rough form, in phrases rather than sentences, but well researched, and interspersed with notes to me.

I then organize the material into sentences, sequences of ideas, paragraphs, and sections. Along the way, I add the headings, introductions, descriptions, closings, metaphors, local color, or anything else that might seem needed. My goal is to round out the text by elaborating on the issues in an accessible writing style. As a writer with many years of experience contributing ideas to health-related subjects, I add reflections that are relevant but require no medical training; some call for research on my part, but many are speculative. I tend to contribute the most content where topics are more general and abstract—for example, comparisons between medical paradigms.

It's a great honor to partake in the creation of a work that has the potential to transform as many lives as this one does. I like to think that a male coauthor can offer a balanced perspective on women's sexual-health concerns—and add extra insights on issues that affect men the most. As always, I hope my writing, ideas, illustrations, and graphics will do justice to Laurie's work, and serve to broadcast part of her amazing gift as a healer to the many thousands of readers who deserve it.

Best wishes,
Alex Steelsmith

Disclaimer: This book contains many self-help treatments and resources, but for serious health issues readers should seek treatment from an appropriate health-care professional. None of the treatments, recommendations, and protocols described in this book are intended as substitutes for qualified professional advice from a licensed naturopathic physician or practitioner of Chinese medicine.

INTRODUCTION

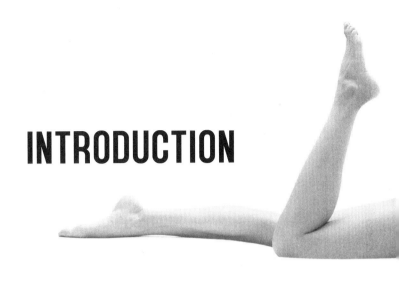

The Promise of Passion:
Embracing New Beginnings

"No journey carries one far unless, as it extends into the world around us, it goes an equal distance into the world within."

— LILLIAN SMITH, *THE JOURNEY*

Imagine this: You're 20 years older than you are now, and head over heels in love with the man of your dreams. You have the energy to exercise every day, take long walks, and entertain or go out every weekend. Your sexual vitality is so high that you often enjoy making love three or four times a week. You feel perpetually optimistic, deeply happy, and radiantly healthy. Isn't this how you want to be 20 years from now—and at every other time in your life?

Are You Ready for a Sexual Power Surge?

If you're looking for a way to recharge your sexual energy and at the same time transform your overall health at any age, then this is the book you've been waiting for. The first work of its kind devoted to optimizing women's sexual health with the techniques of natural medicine, it covers a wealth of ancient secrets and modern methods for increasing your libido, including specific tips, advice, and practical information that has never been made widely available. The information in these pages empowers you to make changes in your life that will benefit you every day.

This book also directly addresses your concerns if you long for more intimacy in your life, but feel you just don't have the energy to rekindle the flame of passion. If this is your experience, you're not alone: an estimated 40 million American women struggle with diminished libido. According to some sources, statistics show that up to 63 percent of women experience some degree of sexual dysfunction during their lives, and low sexual desire is their most frequent concern.

You may experience low libido at any time in your life; it happens to women in their 20s and 30s, as well as those in midlife and their senior years. Perhaps you wake up one morning and realize that *sex* has become just another word. You know you're missing something, because you vividly recall the rich connotation those three letters used to hold for you—how they once conveyed a sense of energy, mystery, and excitement, and seemed to conduct an almost palpable electrical charge. You may wonder what happened, and how such an alluring word could ever have lost its luster. Are you often more interested in watching television than making love? Did you somehow sublimate all your desire into accomplishments, friends, or family? Are you allotted only a limited supply of sexual energy to spend in your lifetime—a certain karmic quota—and can it be that you've already exhausted yours?

For many who practice conventional medicine, the answer is yes: your libido wanes, they may tell you, as your hormones change over the course of your life. This book invites you to not only question that answer, but disprove it in a hundred ways. It offers a refreshing perspective: you were designed by nature to be a sensual, vibrant, energetic woman for your entire life. Your sexuality changes through time, but that doesn't mean loss; a waning libido can be a symptom of underlying imbalances—and opportunities for greater balance and sexual health. The truth is that at any age you can take charge of your sexuality and restore your libido, and *sex* can once again convey a sense of mystery, power, and passion in your life. As much as ever before, you can experience how it feels for your sexual energy to flourish, and know what it means to treasure pleasure.

Women's sexual-health needs clearly aren't being adequately met by conventional medicine. You see images of female sexuality projected everywhere in the media and advertising, yet if you need reliable advice on how to naturally cultivate sexual health, you may have nowhere to turn. At times in your life, your hormonal shifts result in physical and emotional changes that can dramatically affect your sexuality, but many physicians may overlook key sexual-health issues, or don't know exactly what to tell women who need help in certain areas. Some women may be misdiagnosed as having *anhedonia*—the inability to experience pleasure—when in fact their pleasure potential is alive and well, and begging for the right treatment in order to be released. Our medical establishment perpetuates the notion that women should take conventional hormones, at some point in their lives, for many issues, and especially for reduced libido. But many women have legitimate concerns about hormones' side effects, which include increased risk of heart disease and breast cancer.

One of the central ideas of this book—that your capacity for sexual pleasure and your overall health are profoundly connected—isn't new. Many have alluded to it down through the ages. The idea appears in ancient Chinese medicine, which holds that sex is essential for health, and in some Western writings: in the 1900s, the controversial psychologist Wilhelm Reich was considered a pioneer by many for his work exploring the relationship between sexuality and health—although 21st-century women may find some of his ideas eccentric or difficult to grasp. Today, we have the advantage of a large body of accumulated scientific research to support the thesis that sexual pleasure and health are inextricably linked.

As we did research for this book, it was surprising to find how much of its material hasn't yet been clearly elucidated or extensively published. This is, after all, the topic of *sex;* you tend to assume that it's all been said before. Yet many priceless pearls of information—including even some specific aphrodisiacs—haven't been made accessible in a reader-friendly way. (It seems hardly possible, for example, that everyone doesn't already know all about such natural wonders as cordyceps, epimedium, catuaba, muira puama, and damiana, to name a few.) This book puts at your fingertips everything you need to naturally enhance your sexuality and take control of your sexual health in ways that will forever change your life. You can use it as your personal guide to *what really works*—the most effective tools and techniques on the subject, some handed down from one generation to the next for millennia, and others discovered in modern times.

Although this book charts a general course you can follow, your personal journey to great sex is like no one else's. As Chapter 3 points out, not every woman's sexuality neatly fits the "sexual response cycle" often used as the blueprint for sizing up sexual health. This book brings together all the brightest stars among natural sex-enhancement methods, but you'll need to navigate your own itinerary through the galaxy of information it offers, find what works best for you, and select a unique niche in your constellation of choice. The number of ways to arrive at great sex may be, like the number of stars in the universe, in the *sex*tillions.

Your Great Sex Journey: Using This Book to Most Effectively Enhance Your Sexuality

To get the most out of this book, we recommend you read it as a whole. You might be tempted to skip ahead to specific sex-enhancing pearls, or zero in on natural solutions to particular sexual-health issues. But some of the most valuable advice in these pages will be applied more effectively if you absorb the book in its entirety and use it as a vehicle for a larger sexual awakening. Certain aphrodisiacs that you'll discover, for instance, aren't apt to work wonders if you haven't utilized the many other libido-boosting tools you'll find in different chapters. If you glean all of the secrets in this book, their cumulative effects can be far-reaching. You may realize many ways to enhance your sexual wellness that you weren't aware of, some of which could be of great relevance to you now—or at a later time in your life.

This book is composed of two main parts, each with its own emphasis:

- In **Part I**, which consists of Chapters 1 through 4, you'll explore a wide range of tools and techniques for enhancing your sexuality, examine the essential cornerstones you need to create a sturdy underpinning for your sexual health, and look at the important roles of your sex organs and hormones.

- In **Part II**—Chapters 5 through 8—you'll discover an array of other means and "new dimensions" you can pursue to enhance not only your own sexuality, but your partner's as well.

Let's take a closer look at the chapter-by-chapter benefits you'll find in these pages:

— We launch our journey in **Chapter 1** by exploring the powerful influence of your mind and spirit on your sexual health. We open with this topic because your mental and spiritual well-being is crucial for creating the foundation you need for a healthy libido, and may be the single most consequential factor in your ability to achieve great sex. Your mind, after all, gives you the power of choice—and your ability to make healthy choices, and act on them, will determine the extent of the benefits you gain from everything you discover in this book. Your mind can open any door, make any choice, and make anything possible.

Chapter 1 begins by looking at the intimate bond between your sexual health and your overall health, and the vital role your mental well-being plays; a healthy mind not only enables you to enjoy sex by freeing you from restrictive emotions and mental states, but can also positively promote your capacity for passion and pleasure in a plethora of ways. This chapter reveals connections between your brain chemistry, the feelings and states of mind you experience when you're in love, and your sexuality and erotic desires. You'll also explore ways of using the power of your mind to create and preserve a strong relationship and a healthy sex life, the physiological basis for your mind's ability to transform your sexuality, links between your sexuality and self-esteem, and more.

— With the vast power of your mind in mind, we continue building on your sexual-health foundation in **Chapter 2** by exploring a way of life that allows you to fully manifest your sexuality. Without this lifestyle, great sex may be a remote possibility; with it, you can reach the heights of sexual satisfaction you're meant to experience. This chapter gives you the solid foundation you need to nourish a dynamic libido with natural step-by-step methods—including wholesome lifestyle choices you can make every day, nutritional supplements, and tips from both ancient Chinese and contemporary Western natural medicine. You'll explore connections between your sexuality and exercise, and you'll gather insights to keep you jazzed about the potential of exercise to rejuvenate your health and sexual energy.

You may be surprised to discover that your ability to detoxify can also revitalize your sexuality. In Chapter 2, we'll explore how you can use detoxification to cleanse your body of impurities that may be hampering your health and limiting your libido—including simple steps you can take to purge your immediate environment of hidden toxins. You'll find a special 21-day dietary cleanse for stimulating your well-being and giving you a sexual-health makeover. When you free yourself from harmful foods, toxins, and other wellness inhibitors, you may feel sexier, healthier, and more alive than ever before.

— Once your "sex-enhancing lifestyle" ducks are all in a row, you'll be primed for **Chapter 3**, which focuses on the centerpiece of your sexuality: your pelvis and sexual organs. For all the pivotal roles this area of your body can play—from sexual pleasure, menstruation, and procreation to supporting your bladder and other vital organs—it deserves extra attention. You'll explore the wondrous, elegant anatomy of your pelvis and sexual organs, and what you most need to know to keep them in peak form. You'll delve into your multidimensional capacity for sexual pleasure, what happens in your body during arousal and orgasm, and the variety of ways a woman can have an orgasm—including the "se-cret" type of orgasm many are unaware of.

In Chapter 3 we'll also explore your "sexual chi" and exercises to increase your pleasure potential and pelvic strength. You'll discover many ways of enhancing your sexuality by overcoming common sexual-health challenges that may arise at some point in your lifetime, including notorious sex spoilers like vaginal dryness, painful menstrual cramps, vaginitis, incontinence, urinary tract infections, pelvic pain, and other conditions. You'll explore a wide range of natural self-help solutions to these challenges—herbs, supplements, food-as-medicine wisdom, natural estrogen creams and hormones, vaginal suppositories, Chinese remedies, acupressure techniques, and other invaluable alternatives to conventional approaches. (At times in this book, "self-help" includes knowing what's available when it comes to certain prescription items, what to ask your doctor for, and how to find the right practitioner in the first place. You'll uncover information an M.D. isn't likely to tell you, but which may be imperative for you to know about in order to find a practitioner who will prescribe what you need.)

— When you discover how much you can do to enhance your sexuality by understanding your hormones—the magical chemicals that shape your libido, health, and practically everything you do—it can make a vast difference in your life. In **Chapter 4,** you'll explore your six most sex-influential hormones, and why keeping them in harmony nurtures your health; gives you energy and vitality; bolsters your zest for life; and helps you feel compassionate, grounded, sexy, stimulated, and empowered on a daily basis. In addition, you'll discover how you can evaluate your hormones and determine if they're healthy or out of balance.

In Chapter 4 you'll also find out how to enhance your sexuality by solving hormone-related imbalances you may encounter at various times in your life, such as diminished sex drive, PMS, heavy menstrual bleeding, adrenal and thyroid issues, infertility, and midlife changes. You'll discover an abundance of natural methods you can use to re-create balance and build your libido—many of them simple measures that allow you to treat yourself effectively without drugs or synthetic hormones—including lifestyle and dietary techniques, bioidentical hormone replacement therapy, supplements, acupressure, herbal remedies, and other gems from natural medicine. You'll also discover how you can improve your body's flow of "Heavenly Water" (the term used by ancient Chinese health practitioners for a woman's menstrual flow), and explore the delightful perspective Chinese medicine offers on hormonal changes you experience over the course of your life.

— In a health-care system dominated by pharmaceutical corporations intent on pushing drugs like Viagra, there's little knowledge of your natural alternatives for sexual enhancement (and even less inclination to tell you about them). **Chapter 5**—the one you're not supposed to flip ahead to, but probably will anyway—is chock-full of unique morsels of sex-enhancing information that can transform your libido in ways no drug can. You'll discover how to get the most out of the world's best natural aphrodisiacs, including legendary Chinese herbal formulas that recharge both your sexuality and your overall health. Many of these natural alternatives are, in a sense, your rightful inheritance, since they were passed down to us over the course of centuries. Their tradition lives on, or you wouldn't be holding this book in your hands.

In Chapter 5 you'll also find a wealth of other kinds of aphrodisiacs and libido-enhancers in the form of herbs, flower essences, essential oils, and more. We'll explore the hidden sensual potential of your own body's natural "secret scents," and look at the fascinating possibilities, and erotically charged signals, literally hanging in the air every time you're in the presence of another person. We'll also explore nutritional aphrodisiacs—including sex-stimulating supplements and foods with potential aphrodisiac effects—and name notorious libido-limiting dietary items that you'll want to avoid.

— In **Chapter 6** we broaden our view to include a variety of other natural pleasure-promoting tools and techniques—from modern to ancient, Western to Eastern, and practical to mystical—that may not be considered aphrodisiacs in the traditional sense, but have aphrodisiac-like qualities. You'll explore a wide selection of moistening and stimulating sensual lubricants, compare products, and find tips on what to look for and what to avoid. You'll also discover the eroticizing effects of acupressure techniques, pelvic self-massage, tantric practices for focusing and expanding your sexual energy, and vaginal strengtheners and releasers, including exercises taught to women centuries ago in China for heightening sexual ecstasy.

With its exploration of both modern and time-honored sensual enhancers, Chapter 6 includes sexual secrets that were readily available to your forebears but are typically off the radar of present-day conventional doctors, who are trained primarily in the use of drugs. Some of the natural sex-enhancers mentioned—particularly those you'll find later in the chapter—can be thought of, like the traditional aphrodisiacs in Chapter 5, as your natural heritage, carefully preserved, handed down over many generations, and bequeathed to you. By using them to enhance your sexuality, you become the heir to some very long traditions, and a living legacy of their effectiveness and staying power.

— We take a different tack in **Chapter 7**, which explores your sexual health in a relationship, and the multitude of ways your partner's sexuality can affect you. In an intimate relationship, your two libidos share a common interface—the realm where your two sexual energies meet and become conjoined—and your sexual health, to a degree, becomes mutual. Enhancing *his* sexuality can benefit yours, and conditions that compromise his sexual health can take a toll on your own. The more you know about supporting his sexual well-being and the specific sexual-health issues he may face during his life, the more you can strengthen your relationship and support your own sexuality.

With this in mind, in Chapter 7 you'll dive into a diversity of important male sexual-health issues. We'll explore natural libido-enhancement methods for your partner, including herbal aphrodisiacs, nutritional supplements, and foods, as well as common conditions that can present challenges for his sexuality. You'll discover natural solutions for erectile dysfunction, and look at the role of drugs like Viagra, their side effects, and how they can affect relationship dynamics. We'll explore low testosterone in detail—its potential effects on your relationship, testing methods, and natural solutions (including bioidentical testosterone treatment) that can benefit you both immeasurably. You'll also gain insights into andropause (male menopause); your partner's hormonal transitions; prostate-gland issues; and a common cause of diminished sexual sensitivity in men, including how it can affect a woman during sex, and what can be done about it.

— In **Chapter 8**, as we near our journey's completion, we'll look back at the previous chapters from a different perspective, and explore ways you can apply what you discover in this book to create lasting changes in your life and make great sex your destiny. Along with an overview of the book's key themes, this chapter includes your "call to action"—a rallying cry of the essential steps you can take to enhance your sexual energy and vitality with natural tools and techniques. Chapter 8 also reaffirms your power to keep making choices that generate your sexual health and well-being, and the Afterword that follows offers closing reflections on the bright future in store for your sexuality.

What Is Natural Medicine, and How Can It Help You Have Great Sex?

Since this book is about how you can achieve great sex *naturally,* it reveals many connections between your sexual health and what's natural. The ancient link between nature and sex is embedded in the English language; the words *nature, gender,* and *genital* all derive from the same Indo-European root. What do we mean by *natural?* In this book, the word is often used in reference to lifestyle choices you can make, and generally means "in accordance with your body's inherent ability to continually re-create your health." As you'll discover, countless decisions you make every day can enhance your natural capacity for great health—and great sex.

The terms *natural health* and *natural medicine,* as used in this book, are based on the principles of naturopathic medicine, which holds the answers to the sexual-health issues of many women. Founded in the 19th century, naturopathic medicine is widely considered America's original and most highly developed tradition of natural health care, and the best example of integrative or holistic medicine. With its focus on creating health rather than merely eliminating disease, and on using methods to stimulate the healing power of nature—your body's innate capacity for maintaining and restoring health—naturopathic medicine strives to avoid drugs with potentially harmful side effects.

Naturopathic medicine sees symptoms as red flags that your body, in its wisdom, gives you to indicate that something needs to change—its way of trying to reestablish a natural balance—rather than indications that you need pharmaceutical medication. If you experience headaches, for example, it isn't because you suffer from an aspirin deficiency. While drugs often suppress symptoms without addressing their underlying causes, the goal of naturopathic medicine is to treat the deeper causes and bring your body back into balance. The most natural, least toxic methods are always used first, and pharmaceutical medicines, surgery, and other invasive techniques may be recommended only as last resorts. There's a time and place for drugs, and they can be lifesaving, but statistically they're also among the leading causes of death in the United States. Natural treatments, on the other hand, are clearly much safer; statistics reveal, for example, that the number of annual deaths in the U.S. caused by vitamins and antioxidants (which can also be lifesaving, in less obvious ways) is virtually zero.

The naturopathic approach considers every aspect of your health, including physical, nutritional, environmental, mental, emotional, and spiritual factors. The emphasis is on lifestyle and prevention—keeping your body strong, and your immunity in good condition through diet, exercise, detoxification, stress management, natural hormones, mental and emotional support, nontoxic alternatives to environmental chemicals, and much more. Naturopathic medicine is all about your choices and your role as a free agent, capable of shaping your own health destiny. *You* have the power to make wise choices that supply every cell in your body with what it needs to function optimally, and you also have the power to remove obstacles to your well-being. This book provides you with many naturopathic treasures you can use to make choices everywhere in your life that will revitalize both your health and your libido. (To learn more about naturopathic medicine, and how to find a doctor trained in natural medicine, see Appendix B.)

Some of the natural health secrets you'll find in this book are drawn from other healing traditions, most notably Chinese medicine. Like naturopathic medicine, this uses natural, nontoxic means; places great emphasis on diet; and considers every feature of your body, mind, and spirit, including environmental factors and behavior patterns. For millennia, Chinese medicine has also emphasized prevention; one of its most revered texts, *The Medical Rules of the Yellow Emperor,* from the 3rd century B.C., compares waiting until you have a health problem and then treating it to waiting until you're thirsty and then digging a well.

Chinese medicine is based on the concept of *chi,* or life force, which courses through your body, brings you vitality and well-being, causes growth and transformation, and protects you from foreign invaders like toxins and bacteria. If you keep your chi abundant, you'll be vigorous and healthy; but if your chi becomes deficient or "stuck," you'll be vulnerable to pain and illness. Your chi comes, in part, from the food you eat and air you breathe; you can influence it with your diet, herbs, exercise, and other life-style choices. And since chi runs through your body in channels known as meridians, you can affect its flow by pressing on acupressure points along your meridians. In this book, you'll discover many ways you can strengthen your chi and enhance your sexual energy with lifestyle choices and acupressure.

Also important in Chinese medicine are the forms of chi known as *yin* and *yang*—opposing forces found throughout nature that shape one another and interact continually. Yin is often represented by feminine sexual energy, darkness, the earth, inwardness, and cold; and yang by masculine sexual energy, light, the sky, outwardness, and heat. Wholeness is achieved whenever yin and yang are joined harmoniously; you're healthy, and your sexual energy can function optimally, when you balance the two in your body, mind, and spirit. In the pages ahead, you'll discover numerous ways of balancing your yin and yang energy to enhance your sexuality.

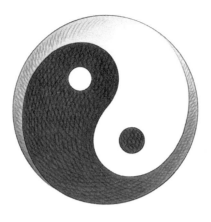

The traditional symbol of yin and yang.

Great Love, Naturally

Anyone can go through the act of sex and appear, on the surface, to have "great sex." But great sex involves something *greater* than great sex. It's about your longing for love and your desire to be whole. You live in the world of your individual mind and body, yet you yearn for the loving connection to another. Sex is your most primal form of reaching out, touching, joining, receiving, giving, sharing, and expressing love. It's at the root of your existence; central to who you are; and integral to your innermost desires, passions, and attractions. The expression of love through sex can give you a sense of being "one," not only with another human but with the universe—transporting you to a state of blissful interconnectedness that, perhaps for just a few fleeting moments, seems eternal.

That's why this book, although it's about sex, is also about much *more* than sex. One of the great secrets about sexual energy is that it's not just for between the sheets. Your sexuality isn't only a matter of genital pleasure, intercourse, and orgasm; research shows that sex activates many of your other physical, cognitive, and emotional capacities. Your sexual energy affects your entire life, touching every dimension of your being. This is reflected in Chinese medicine, which sees your sexual energy as indistinguishable from the vital force that brings potent healing effects to all parts of your body. Your sexuality lies at the core of your life energy, in the wellspring of your creativity and spirit.

This is the greater meaning of "great sex," and what this book is all about. You can use the information gathered in these pages not only to recharge your libido and electrify your sexuality, but also as a way of tapping into the power of your sexual energy to light up your life on all levels. By enhancing your sexual well-being—an essential component of your happiness—you can transform your world. This is why, if you incorporate what you discover in this book into your life, you may find that your partner, friends, or co-workers notice quantum leaps in the amount of energy, confidence, and *joie de vivre* that you exude.

When we refer to sex as "making love," we imply that it literally creates love. The phrase illuminates our intuitive awareness that sex can manifest the strongest possible state of emotional bonding and unity; we *know* that real eroticism engenders intense compassion and empathy. Sex and love are inseparable, it seems, even linguistically; the words *libido* and *love* share a common ancestor.

By expanding your capacity for sexual union through the natural means described in this book, you can liberate the formidable influence of love in your life more fully. Love repairs relationships, changes cultures, moves mountains, and makes the world go 'round, but sex without it does none of these. To paraphrase the famous saying: without love, it is nothing.

Just as sex makes love, love makes sex better; it is your most powerful aphrodisiac. Intriguing research on sexual pleasure and the brain's emotional center suggests that orgasms may be more euphoric when people are in love.

This is a multifaceted book; sex, like love, is a many-splendored thing. But while the chapters ahead give you a wide assortment of tools you can use to achieve great sex—and many involve physical methods for enhancing your libido—it's important to remember that great sex can be a natural consequence of great intimacy. Paradoxically, you may find that the greatest sex derives not from focusing on whether you have the greatest sex, but from focusing on whether you have the greatest *love*.

PART I

GETTING IN BALANCE

The Secrets to Creating Your Ultimate Sexual Health

CHAPTER 1

EXPANDING YOUR SEXUAL POTENTIAL

The Power of Your Mind and Spirit

"The focused human mind is the most powerful instrument in the universe."

— JILL BOLTE TAYLOR, *MY STROKE OF INSIGHT*

Great sex is your birthright; you came into being as the result of orgasm, and your body is perfectly designed for sexual pleasure. You have specialized receptors in your brain, vagina, and clitoris—and throughout your physiology—that serve no other purpose than to give you sensual satisfaction. But even though you were born with the potential for great sex, it's not a given. You have to nurture your capacity for it, allow it time to grow and flourish, and nourish it with care and loving attention.

Your capacity for sexual pleasure is intimately connected to every aspect of your health. To enjoy sex, you need a healthy mind and body, freedom from pain and discomfort, and the energy to act on your desires. Of course, you won't be likely to have great sex if you're chronically ill, tired, depressed, feeling burned-out, struggling with difficult sexual issues, or harboring negative feelings about sex.

But the relationship between your sexuality and your health is far more dynamic than the obvious correlation between your ability to experience erotic sensations and your overall well-being. There are myriad connections between your capacity for pleasure and countless choices you make every day. Everything about your lifestyle—including your state of mind, what you eat, how you exercise, and how efficiently you eliminate toxins—can affect your capacity for sexual pleasure. Over time, you can fully manifest your potential for great sex with the right choices, or you can diminish it with unhealthy ones. Just as people who let their health go for many years may lose the natural function of an organ or system, it's possible to gradually undermine your natural capacity for sexual gratification with lifestyle choices that relentlessly torpedo your libido. Great sex can be yours for as long as you live, but you have to choose it again and again with a lifestyle that supports it. The choice is yours; choose it or lose it.

Not only does abundant mental and physical health increase your capacity to enjoy sex, but sex, in turn, gives you many health benefits. In fact, a climax a day keeps the doctor away: sex reduces stress, burns calories, increases your circulation (bringing nutrients and fresh oxygen to your tissues), and releases "feel-good" oxytocin and endorphins, as well as prolactin (which promotes calmness and reduced blood pressure). And sex has many other potential benefits as well: it may help strengthen your immunity; aid in pain relief (including that of menstrual cramps and migraines); lower the risk of heart attacks, endometriosis, and preterm deliveries in pregnant women; promote consistent menstrual cycles; stimulate your vagina's natural lubrication; and prevent urinary incontinence. Some research also suggests a link between frequency of sex and longevity.

Health and sex are, in a sense, mutually reinforcing: the greater your health, the greater your capacity to enjoy sex; and the more you enjoy sex, the greater your health. Health makes you sexy, and sex makes you healthy!

In Part I of this book, you'll explore the four cornerstones essential for nurturing your potential to have great sex: your mind and spirit, diet, exercise habits, and ability to detoxify. We begin with your mind and spirit because they're uniquely pivotal; all of the choices that influence your sexual destiny emerge from your mind, after all. Through the power of choice making, your mind will be the crucial determining factor for every one of the tools you'll discover in this book for building your health and libido. Many of the benefits you stand to gain will be for naught if your mind and spirit aren't healthy.

Your state of mind is also connected to your capacity for sexual pleasure in innumerable other ways. Not only does your ability to fully enjoy sex require a healthy mind and spirit, the clarity of consciousness to pursue your passions, and freedom from unhealthy emotions, but every state of mind you experience can have profound effects on your physiology and resistance to disease, as well as your potential for great sex. Your capacity for sexual pleasure is inseparable from your mind—in a sense, pleasure is nothing more than the *awareness* of pleasure—which may make your mind the ultimate measure of pleasure.

In this chapter you'll explore ways in which you can engage your mind and spirit to enhance your health and change your life—especially in order to create or maintain a healthy love relationship and a fulfilling sex life. By tapping into the strength of your mind and spirit with the thoughts, tools, and techniques in the following pages, you can vastly expand your possibilities for enjoying great sex, naturally.

Your Brain: Sex, Love, and Limbic Linkage

Your mind and spirit are related to your physical brain, and thus in order to most effectively use the power of your mind and spirit to enhance your libido, it helps to begin by knowing how your brain can affect your sexuality. Let's take a look at your brain health, and some critical connections between your brain chemistry, your sexual health, and the intense emotions you can feel in a relationship.

All of the steps you'll discover in the next chapter for building the foundation of your general health and supporting your sexuality with diet, exercise, and detoxification also support your *brain* health; every feature of your Great Sex Lifestyle is brain boosting. At the same time, improving your brain health gives you additional paybacks everywhere in your life. Neurons, neurotransmitters, and hormones play key roles in all your thoughts, moods, and feelings—including your ability to feel love, sexual attraction, pleasure, and orgasm. And as your most powerful sex organ, your brain contains everything you think about sex.

Sex, in turn, affects your brain by releasing the important brain chemicals oxytocin and endorphins, which can improve your moods and elevate your tolerance for pain. And research shows that when you have an orgasm, the area of your brain that controls fear and anxiety is temporarily disengaged, which potentially benefits your nervous system.

The sex-related brain chemicals released in your body can vary, depending on which phase of a relationship you're in. When you first fall in love and during the early stages of a romance, you're more likely to be bathed by the sex hormones estrogen and testosterone (this is true for both women and men) and the neurotransmitters adrenaline, serotonin, and dopamine. Increased adrenaline can elevate your heart rate and cause you to perspire when you think of your new love. A rise in serotonin may explain, in part, your preoccupation with thinking about him; research shows that serotonin levels of new sexual partners can be similar to those of people with obsessive-compulsive disorder. And increased dopamine can incite strong sensations of pleasure that have effects on your brain similar to cocaine (but without harming your body), giving you surges of energy, reducing your need for food and sleep, and stimulating your capacity for focused attention—especially the attention you give to your new relationship.

After the initial stages of love, two hormones appear to play vital roles in the development of long-term attachment: vasopressin and oxytocin. Research indicates that vasopressin, which is released after sex, promotes bonding and devotedness. And oxytocin, the "intimacy hormone" released by both women and men during orgasm, also promotes bonding and deepens feelings of attachment, especially after sex. And your bond grows stronger, research suggests, with each act of lovemaking. In the realm of your hormones, as in so many others, sex connects; the more you make love, the more love you make.

As you continue a relationship, gradual physiological changes occur in a portion of your brain called the *limbic system*—the "emotional center," developed in your infancy and childhood.

Your limbic system helps you form attachments to others, and plays a part in your ability to find another person attractive and fall in love. During a long-term relationship, you become "limbically connected" with your partner; both of your limbic systems lay down new neural cells, in effect shifting your brain anatomies in response to interactions with one another over time.

Your capacity for limbic linkage explains, to some extent, the depths of feeling and commitment you can experience in a long-term relationship, and why you may feel at times as if your identity becomes fused with your partner's. As Thomas Lewis, M.D., wrote of limbic connectedness in *A General Theory of Love:* "Who we are and who we become depends, in part, on whom we love." The force of limbic bonding is one reason why it can take years to recover from the loss of a long-term relationship; your limbic system's circuitry is without its "other half," the specific person it had formed for.

Using Your Mind to Build and Preserve a Healthy Relationship

Being aware of your brain's natural physiological tendencies can help you understand thoughts and emotions you experience around issues of love and sex, but your mind and spirit are greater than the sum of your brain's cells, chemical messengers, and physical components. Intimate relationships are profoundly spiritual and emotional, and can't be reduced to these factors alone. It remains largely mysterious that your evolving mind and spirit can connect with another evolving mind and spirit, love deeply, commit to sharing yourself over time, and express love through the physical medium of sex.

At the same time, by harnessing the power of your mind, you can enhance your natural ability to live in the mystery of love. Let's look at some important ways you can use your mind to build and maintain a strong love relationship and a healthy sex life. All of them can be put to good use in conjunction with the other tools and techniques you'll explore in the chapters ahead. While you're busy building your libido and your overall health, you can be relationship building at the same time!

— **Creating time.** It may seem obvious that you need quality time alone with your partner, without the intrusions of the world, to have a dynamic, supportive love relationship and experience great sex. Yet many people seem to forget to find time for relationship nurturing, perhaps because they feel caught up in a culture that places higher priorities on other things. One of the secrets of partners who evolve together over many years, and continue to love one another and enjoy a healthy sex life, is creating time to spend together and fully appreciate one another—which means more than just making time for sex.

In the modern world, many couples are separated on a daily basis by work and other responsibilities, but with the strength of your mind, you can turn this to your advantage. Humans are sometimes distinguished from other animals because of our unusual capacity for delayed gratification; we can imagine enjoyable experiences well in advance, and doing so may enhance pleasure. This pertains not only to simply spending time with your partner, but also to sex: in a sense, you can *enhance in advance*. If you have to wait, let anticipation increase gratification.

— **Communication and sex.** For many couples in healthy relationships, there are profound connections between the quality of their communication and the quality of their sex life. When you share intimate thoughts and feelings with one another on a daily basis over time—not merely discussions of household functions, paying bills, or material possessions, but your most personal issues—you continue to grow and evolve together, and you become closer in every way, including sexually. It's almost as if the natural give-and-take of good communication, along with all of its other relationship-building benefits, has an added aphrodisiac effect.

— **Sexual trust.** Building an emotionally safe, solid relationship can be critical to the health of your partnership and your sex life. Many women have difficulty achieving orgasm, or even becoming aroused, unless they're in a relationship that allows them to fully let go, trust, and release control. Modern brain research backs this up; brain scans show that during orgasm women— unlike men, who experience stimulation of their "reward" circuitry—have reduced activity in brain areas that govern self-control, moral reasoning, social judgment, and vigilance. Your capacity for pleasure appears to be closely linked with your brain's ability to release inhibition, suspend judgment, and let down your guard, all of which may be possible only when you're in a relationship that feels dependable and secure.

— **Supporting your right brain.** Your brain is *bicameral*, which means it's composed of "two houses," or halves. Each has functions that offer you a different perspective of the world; your left hemisphere is more logical and linear, and your right more intuitive and nonlinear. Many women caught up in the busy world of day-to-day responsibilities function highly from their left brain but have lost touch with the holistic, nurturing potential of their right brain.

In *My Stroke of Insight,* Jill Bolte Taylor describes how, after being trained to rely heavily on her left hemisphere as a brain scientist, she experienced a stroke that damaged her left brain and opened her eyes to the workings of her right hemisphere. During her recovery, while her right brain dominated, she experienced blissful sensations of love, compassion, peace, and interconnectedness with all things. Her descriptions are reminiscent of the teachings of Eastern religions and ancient meditation practices on becoming "one" with the cosmos.

Tapping into the right side of your brain can help you maintain a balanced life, improve your sense of well-being, and nurture your capacity for a healthy intimate relationship. It can also get you in touch with "the sensuality mentality"—your natural ability to experience all the joys of loving sexual union. Your two-sided brain is exquisitely designed to allow you full awareness of sexual pleasure; it is, if you will, your great sex duplex. But for many women, it's the power of the right brain that allows them to experience pleasure while disengaging from other mental activities, in a sense liberating sexuality from intellectuality.

You don't need to have a stroke to cultivate the potential of your right brain; you can stimulate its neuronal circuitry with virtually any activity that gives you a temporary reprieve from tasks governed by your left brain and engages your natural intuitive powers. In addition to meditation, examples include art, music, dance, yoga, and many forms of spontaneity and play.

You Can Change Your Mind, Whenever You Want

The quotation at the beginning of this chapter says it all: your "mind is the most powerful instrument in the universe." You can do practically anything you put your mind to, and you can put your mind to practically *anything*. Your thoughts influence your feelings and behavior from one moment to the next, so at any point in time you can change your thoughts and change your life. As Louise Hay has written in *Heal Your Body*, "by changing our thinking patterns, we can change our experiences." Your conscious intentions and beliefs can shape your destiny, and you can choose happiness, health, beneficial relationships, love, and sexual fulfillment. The most important step you can take to enhance your sexuality is to consciously choose a set of thoughts and beliefs that will create, not negate, great sex—in short, a *credo for your libido*.

This is underscored by an understanding of how your brain functions. One of its most wonderful qualities is *plasticity*—its capacity to be malleable and changeable. By consciously altering the thoughts that dominate your life, you redirect your perceptions. Over time, this changes neurochemicals released, and reshapes your brain's circuitry by creating new nerve tracks and altering your very cells. By choosing new thoughts, you can thus "rewire" your brain, override old patterns of thinking and behavior, and ultimately transform your relationship to the world and to your sexual partner.

The key to choosing new, more health-affirming thoughts is becoming conscious of your present thinking patterns and choices and how they may be affecting your health, relationships, or sexuality. By increasing your awareness, you can discover areas where you may be unknowingly working *against* yourself—for example, with thoughts that subvert your health or sabotage a relationship—and replace them with thoughts you need in order to make better choices. As Wayne Dyer says in his book *There's a Spiritual Solution to Every Problem,* it's a matter of keeping your focus on what you want in your life: "If your thoughts are on what you don't want . . . you will act upon those thoughts and more of what you don't want will keep showing up." You're well on your way to achieving a great sex life if you simply keep your eyes on the prize.

Let's look at some do-it-yourself methods you can use to clear your mind and get in touch with the life-altering potential of your thoughts to support a relationship or your sexuality:

— **Making time for change.** This means setting aside quiet times to calmly reflect on your life and examine your thought patterns. It's about using "mental floss" at least once daily to clear your mind of all the accumulated debris and distractions of commercials, television, magazines, computers, e-mail, social media, and cell phones. By getting away from all of the mental chatter, and disconnecting from the potential negativity of anything that might trigger you emotionally, you can concentrate on whatever positive changes you want to generate for your health or your sex life.

— **Affirmations.** You can use positive self-talk—words repeated aloud or in your mind—to free yourself from negative thoughts and focus on your goals. Consistency is helpful; you need sufficient repetition over a period of time for the positive effects of affirmations to permeate your consciousness and bring about changes in your brain. Examples of affirmations include: *I make choices that benefit me, I excel at reaching my goals, I take care of and nurture myself, I choose radiant health, I focus on the positive,* and *I achieve my dreams.* Examples pertaining more directly to your sexuality include: *I fulfill my sexual nature, I'm destined to attain my ultimate sexual satisfaction, My body effortlessly manifests sexual pleasure, I love the expression of my sexual energy, A wonderful, loving relationship happens naturally for me,* and *I can create whatever degree of love and sexual fulfillment I choose.*

If you ever catch yourself having a self-deprecating thought, make a point to assert affirmations that correct it. You can also use affirmations at any other time—for example, while you're stuck in traffic, or waiting for an appointment. They may be particularly effective when you awaken in the morning, and your mind is like a blank canvas. One of my patients—who's not only a strong swimmer but also an exceptionally healthy, loving, and kind person—recently turned 90. Her secret? It turns out that for many years, during her morning swims, she has said to herself, in rhythm with each stroke, *I'm strong, healthy, loving, kind.*

— **Meditation.** Many meditation techniques that focus on breathing can be calming and clarifying, and help you get in touch with your mind and spirit—and their ability to shape your health and sexuality. For starters, try this simple technique: For a few minutes each day, sit comfortably, close your eyes, and consciously inhale by first expanding your stomach to fill your lower lungs and then expanding your chest to fill your upper lungs. Slowly exhale in the same order, first using your stomach to expel air from your lower lungs, then allowing your chest to expel air from your upper lungs. You can enhance this technique by visualizing that you're inhaling life-giving, clear white light, and exhaling gray smoke containing any negative thoughts lingering in your body.

— **Keeping a journal.** Expressing your thoughts in writing is another powerful way of heightening your awareness and focusing your mind and spirit on any changes you want to create for your health and sexuality. The act of physically spelling out your intentions on paper, with its unique reliance on your mind-hand connection, can effectively reroute neural circuits in your brain, redirect your consciousness, and supersede old thoughts. If you keep a journal, it's a good idea to make entries on a regular basis. As with affirmations, you may find that writing first thing in the morning is especially rewarding.

Sex and Your Self-Esteem

Your self-esteem is of paramount importance in creating a strong intimate relationship and a healthy sex life. Your ability to love yourself is a prerequisite to loving another, and self-esteem affects every aspect of your life. Let's look at how you can gauge your self-esteem status, particularly with issues relating to sexuality, and whether you need to improve it.

You may have low self-esteem if you frequently feel sexually inhibited, insecure about your appearance, or ashamed of sexual activity you engage in. Other common indicators include difficulty achieving orgasm (either alone or with a partner), having sex with partners you don't love, or believing that there's something "wrong" with you sexually.

The way you choose your sexual partner can also reveal something about your level of self-esteem. If you have high self-esteem, you're likely to feel attracted to a potential partner who has it as well, and you're also more apt to use the power of your mind to assist you in making a healthy choice. If your self-esteem is low, you may feel drawn to a partner with similar low self-regard, which can be compounded by believing that you don't deserve a better choice. You may also be more prone to "impulse buy" when choosing a partner, with potentially disastrous results; the person you find attractive on the spur of the moment isn't always a wise choice.

Another way to assess the level of your self-esteem is by looking at your behavior patterns once you're in a relationship. The ways in which you interact with your partner can tell you a lot about how you think and feel about yourself. The following is a summary of what your relationship can reveal about your self-esteem quotient. No one factor definitively means you have either high or low self-esteem. These indicators are simply to give you an overall sense of where you stand in your own estimation.

Signs of High Self-Esteem in a Relationship

If you have healthy self-esteem, you communicate honestly with your partner, you openly express your feelings when you need to, and your relationship supports your inner emotional self. You feel a clear sense of your own identity, you have the courage to be yourself, and you're comfortable saying no if you don't want to go along with something your partner wants to do, sexually or otherwise. You bring all aspects of your personality to the relationship and live fully and authentically in the present, as opposed to putting up a facade of who you are.

Another sign of your high self-esteem is that your partner displays all of these same qualities. You love, support, nurture, and respect him just as much as he does you. Your relationship is reciprocal, and you evolve together. It gives both of you a solid base and a constant source of strength from which you can thrive as whole people, pursue your dreams, and maximize your potential as a couple and as individuals. And as two self-esteeming people, you're more likely to experience a healthy sex life.

Signs of Low Self-Esteem in a Relationship

If you have low self-esteem, you may exhibit one of two characteristic behavior patterns in a relationship:

1. In one scenario, you present yourself as a victimized "wounded woman," and give off signals that you need help. You tend to attract men who feel compelled to save you from your predicament—whether that be poor health, personal problems, eating disorders or other addictive behaviors, or professional failings. Although your partner may make valiant efforts to help, you're likely to give him mixed signals and sabotage the relationship with destructive impulses or behaviors, because you're unable to change as long as your self-esteem remains low.

2. The second, more common scenario is almost the opposite. You tend to "lose yourself" in a relationship, sacrificing your needs, emotional security, or even physical safety in an effort to please your partner, conform to his ideas of who you should be, or "rescue" him from difficulties in his life. You may hide parts of yourself that don't support your partner's needs, let go of your dreams, suppress your creativity, or "self-collapse" (disappear emotionally) when conflict arises. You're liable to experience lots of drama in the relationship, with poor communication leading to emotionally volatile outbursts of arguing, stress, and unhappiness, which can be all-consuming and further prevent you from pursuing your goals. You tend to stay in the relationship, even if your partner is verbally or physically abusive, because you're afraid to be alone or believe he couldn't live without you.

In this second scenario, the effects of low self-esteem can be of particular consequence for the quality of your sexual relationship. You may be so focused on your partner's pleasure that it interferes with or negates your own ability to experience pleasure, or be so afraid of disappointing him or being rejected by him that you avoid sex altogether. At times, you may go through the motions of having sex, even though you don't want to, because you believe it will make the relationship work. One way or another, your sexual needs aren't met. Many women in this category exhibit the "chameleon syndrome": they conform to whatever sexual tone is set by their partner. As one 60-year-old told me, "I've had many relationships, but always acquiesced to the sexual needs of the man I was with. I still don't know what my own sexual needs would be if it were up to me." She'd lived through the sexual revolution, yet never allowed herself to experience her own natural sexuality.

In either of the preceding scenarios, your relationship tends to be nonreciprocal; you're not true partners, and the relationship doesn't ultimately help either of you achieve your potential, as your low self-esteem prevents you from being loved for who you are or otherwise gets in the way. And because *you* don't have high self-esteem, your partner may not esteem you either, which can further exacerbate the problem and prevent you from experiencing a healthy sex life.

What to Do If You Need to Build Your Self-Esteem

If you have low self-esteem, the good news is that there are effective ways you can address the condition, rebuild your self-confidence, get past unhealthy sexual patterns, and tap into your highest potential. An in-depth exploration of solutions for low self-esteem is beyond the scope of this book, but the following suggestions can help you to start moving in the right direction:

— **Seek out a therapist.** This may be the single most important step you can take to improve your self-esteem. A good therapist is a catalyst you can use to get where you want to go much more quickly. Therapy can help you identify patterns in your behavior, sexuality, and communication that may undermine your efforts to become a more whole, self-esteeming person. By examining your early relationships with your parents or primary caregivers, you may discover where feelings of low self-worth began. Becoming conscious of your patterns, strengths, and weaknesses allows you to shift your perspective and ultimately change your behavior and your choices.

— **Affirm your worth.** To access your natural ability to be a healthy, vibrant, sexual woman, you first have to realize that you have that potential. True health and beauty come from the inside out; as the saying goes, you're as beautiful as you feel. When you get in touch with your self-esteeming, gorgeous self, you take better care of yourself and you emanate energy that attracts other self-esteeming people. As explained earlier in this chapter, you can change your brain, and your actions, through the potent influence of your thoughts. You can use affirmations to connect with the intuitive, nonlinear power of your right brain, change your beliefs about yourself, and elevate your self-esteem. Examples of affirmations for boosting self-esteem include: *I honor and value myself, I have unlimited worth and potential, I'm beautiful and attractive,* and *I'm worthy of the highest love.*

Conclusion: Keeping the Power of Your Mind in Mind

In this chapter we've considered a diversity of approaches for using your mind and spirit to nourish your natural potential for sexual fulfillment. We've touched on your brain health and how it can affect your sexual energy and the emotions you experience when you're in love. We've also looked at ways you can use your mind to support a relationship, supplant limiting habits of thought, empower your sexuality, and more.

As you move forward with the rest of this book, remember that with your mind—the miraculous entity that gives you the power of choice—you can achieve practically anything. Continually engaging the strength of your mind to keep making healthy choices will inestimably boost your ability to reap the benefits of the many sex-enhancing tips and secrets you'll discover in subsequent chapters. Remaining mindful that mindfulness itself can multiply the potential of every page will transform your life and lead you to vastly greater sexual health.

CHAPTER 2

NURTURING INTIMACY

The Great Sex Lifestyle

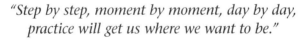

*"Step by step, moment by moment, day by day,
practice will get us where we want to be."*

— Louise Hay, *Empowering Women*

We began the previous chapter with the idea that although sexual pleasure is your natural birthright, you have to nurture your capacity for great sex in order for it to flourish. On one level, your potential for sexual pleasure is connected to your health in obvious ways: to be capable of fully enjoying pleasure, you need a healthy body, the energy to be passionate, and freedom from the distractions and restrictions of illness and suffering. You'll be unlikely to experience great sex if your health is often out of balance, you're constantly dealing with challenging symptoms, or you're frequently exhausted.

On a deeper level, the effects of your health on your sexuality are far more consequential than you may realize at first glance. Countless choices you make every day—every facet of your lifestyle, including, as Chapter 1 explored, even your thoughts—can have direct or indirect long-term repercussions for your capacity for pleasure. The cumulative effects of numerous healthy choices, over the course of months and years, can allow your natural potential for radiant sexual health to thrive. On the other hand, consistent unhealthy choices can gradually reduce your sexual energy and ultimately undercut your capacity for pleasure.

Many people spend their lives somewhere between these two extremes, in a kind of libido limbo, never fully experiencing the sexual gratification they're capable of and unaware of the extent of their birthright to pleasure. If you're in this category, you may be amazed to uncover the power of the gifts you have lying dormant. This power may be only waiting for you to make the right lifestyle choices to allow it to emerge and reveal itself. And in addition, as we pointed out previously, abundant health not only increases your capacity to enjoy sex, but in a "virtuous" cycle, sex gives you many health benefits in return—another reason why becoming healthier can be synonymous with becoming sexier.

Now that we've explored the power of your mind and spirit—the first cornerstone of your sexual health—you'll look at many more ways you can bring out your capacity for great sex with a healthy lifestyle. In this chapter, we'll examine the three other key cornerstones that form the foundation of your sexual health: your diet, your exercise habits, and your ability to efficiently remove toxins from your body. You'll discover many tools and techniques you can use on a daily basis to unlock your hidden potential and maximize your ability to experience your natural inheritance to pleasure.

The Great Sex Diet

Your diet is an area of your life that's completely within your control, and it can have profound effects on your body and its resistance to disease, and on your zest for life. It may even help you fulfill your genetic potential. According to well-known researcher Jeffrey Bland, you can "alter the expression of your genes" with the food you eat. By providing you with high-quality food, the Great Sex Diet gives you the basis for more energy, potentially greater genetic expression, better sex-hormone production, and a more robust sex life.

You can eat only so much at any given time, so you want to choose the most densely nutritious options—high-vitality foods chock-full of essential nutrients. Every bite of every meal is an opportunity to add fuel to your body that will make the most of your health and your pro-libido lifestyle on a cellular level.

Let's look at the basic components of your Great Sex Diet:

— **Choose organic.** There's nothing sexy about eating non-organic food. By choosing organic, in one move you can avoid numerous pesticides; genetically modified organisms (GMOs); fertilizers made with synthetic ingredients or sewage sludge (some fertilizers contain waste treated at sewage plants, and may harbor food-contaminating ingredients); irradiation (nonorganic foods may be irradiated to extend their shelf life, a questionable practice for your health); and antibiotics and growth hormones.

Foods containing GMOs may be, by definition, among the unsexiest edibles in the universe, since they're produced not by normal reproductive processes, but by inserting genetic material from one organism into another, giving foods genetic traits they don't naturally have. Some genetically modified foods contain material that has never been consumed by humans and may pose serious allergy threats or result in antibiotic resistance. An extra word of caution regarding GMOs, particularly if you live in the U.S.: Although GMO foods haven't been adequately tested for safety, the FDA, unlike regulators in many other countries, doesn't require that they be labeled. In the U.S., buying 100 percent organic is the only way to ensure that you aren't consuming GMOs.

— **Enjoy "good" carbohydrates.** Ignore the popular notion that all carbohydrates are bad for you. Eating the right carbohydrates can give your body the sustained, consistent energy it needs to power your muscles, brain, and libido. It's only *simple* carbohydrates that you want to avoid, not complex ones. Simple carbohydrates, like white rice, have little fiber in them; on the other hand, complex carbohydrates, such as brown rice, give you lots of valuable fiber.

19

Fiber is the part of your diet that your body doesn't digest. Along with many other benefits, it keeps you from feeling hungry too soon after a meal and prevents you from experiencing extreme highs and lows in your blood-sugar level. If you have steady blood sugar throughout the day, you have better regulation of your energy (sexual and otherwise), improved mental functioning, and greater feelings of well-being. Typically, the more fiber in a food, the lower its glycemic index—a measurement of how quickly a food converts into sugar in your body—so you want to choose carbohydrates with a low glycemic index.

— **Eat high-quality, lean protein.** Your body, mind, and libido rely on adequate protein to be optimally healthy. Protein serves as a precursor to important neurotransmitters, which, as you'll discover later in this chapter, can be vital for your sexuality. Healthy protein sources include beans and legumes, eggs, nonfat dairy foods, lean chicken and turkey, and low-mercury fish and seafood.

— **Consume omega-3 essential fats, and avoid unhealthy fats.** To function optimally, your entire body, including your sexual organs, needs essential fats—"essential" because your body doesn't produce them, and you have to ingest them in your diet. There are two kinds of essential fats: *omega-3 fats* and *omega-6 fats.* As a rule, you want to increase your intake of omega-3 fats, which have a wide range of health benefits. They assist in maintaining the moisture and health of your vulvar tissues, help with your production of sex hormones, and improve your circulation—including blood flow to your sexual organs, which enhances your ability to feel aroused. Omega-3 fats aren't often consumed in the typical Western diet. They're abundant in fish and flax oils; hemp, chia, and pumpkin seeds; walnuts; and seafood. If you take fish oil as a supplement, the recommended daily dose is an amount containing at least 500 mg of the omega-3 fatty acid EPA (eicosapentaenoic acid) and 300 mg of another omega-3 fatty acid, DHA (docosahexaenoic acid).

Omega-6 fats are found in corn, soy, cottonseed, safflower, and sunflower oils. Most Americans eat far too many omega-6 fats; it's generally recommended that you avoid increasing your omega-6 intake.

Other unsexy fats to minimize in your diet include saturated fats found in beef, pork, lamb, turkey, chicken, and whole-milk products like cheese and butter. It's best to steer clear of all hydrogenated fats (also known as trans-fatty acids), which are found in margarines, some candy bars, and many processed foods. These fats can obstruct female (as well as male) sex-hormone production; research also shows that these fats promote hardening of the arteries, which can contribute to erectile dysfunction in men.

— **Eat lots of fruit and vegetables.** By providing you with life-sustaining nutrition, vegetables support your sexuality. They should make up at least a third of your diet, and you should eat a minimum of ten servings a day whenever possible. Fruit is another important part of your Great Sex Diet, but keep in mind that it also contains a lot of simple sugar, so you may need to limit your intake. Avoid watermelon, cantaloupe, and mangoes; they're high in fruit sugar, which can cause rapid increases, followed by steep drops, in your blood-sugar level—not good for your health or your sexual energy. In the pages ahead, we'll explore some fruits and fruit juices that are exceptionally conducive to your overall well-being and sexual health.

— **Drink plenty of filtered water.** Keeping yourself well hydrated enhances your sexuality by helping to maintain your body's self-moisturizing function, which includes your natural production of vaginal lubrication. When you're aroused, your vagina's ability to produce ample lubrication—potentially critical for your sexual pleasure—depends in part on your prior fluid intake.

Supplements to Reinforce Your Great Sex Diet

You can guarantee that you're getting the nutrients you need to support your body and your sexuality by backing up your diet with the right vitamin and mineral supplements. No matter how carefully you eat, you may not always get all the necessary nutrients—because of seasonal unavailability of foods, depletion of minerals in the soil from certain farming practices (which can reduce nutrient content in your foods), fluctuations in your individual bodily needs and stress level, your exposure to particular health challenges (including contagious illnesses and environmental contaminants), and many other factors. The best way to ensure that you're getting a baseline of vitamins and minerals to meet your needs is by taking the following daily supplements:

— **Multivitamin.** The important ingredients to look for in your multivitamin supplement are vitamins C, D, E, B_2, B_6, and B_{12}, as well as thiamine, niacin, folate, biotin, pantothenic acid, calcium, magnesium, zinc, selenium, copper, manganese, chromium, molybdenum, beta-carotene, pyridoxal 5-phosphate, potassium, and bioflavonoids. If you use the multivitamin recommended in Appendix C, take two tablets twice daily with food.

— **Antioxidant formula.** The key ingredients you need in your antioxidant formula are vitamin C, coenzyme Q_{10}, alpha lipoic acid, resveratrol, green-tea extract, and n-acetyl l-cysteine. Your multivitamin contains vitamin C, but the additional C in your antioxidant gives you further immune protection and extra assistance in fighting free radicals. If you use the antioxidant formula in Appendix C, take two capsules daily.

— **Bone formula.** The important ingredients in a good bone-support formula are vitamin K, vitamin K_2, magnesium, calcium, boron, and silica. The multivitamin recommended above contains magnesium and calcium, but women need an extra boost of both for additional bone support. If you take the bone formula in Appendix C, the recommended dose is two capsules daily.

The Dynamic Dozen:
Super-Libido Foods to Enhance Your Great Sex Diet

To provide an extra punch to your sex-supportive diet, you'll want to enjoy the following foods and beverages often. These 12 items are recommended because they're unusually rich in nutrients, vitamins, and minerals that can prevent or treat disease, and have unique potential to promote your overall health and sexual well-being. (Most of these aren't usually considered aphrodisiacs;

later in this book, you'll explore specific foods for their aphrodisiac potential.) They're not listed in order of effectiveness—all are powerful as super-libido foods.

1. **Flax.** Flaxseeds are high in friendly omega-3 fats (which, as you've seen, are favorable to your sexual health), decrease inflammation in your body, and may help prevent cancer. Flaxseeds are also loaded with *lignans,* and research shows that high levels of these phytonutrients in your diet can reduce your breast-cancer risk. To enhance your Great Sex Diet, take one tablespoon of flax oil, containing 6,200 mg of omega-3 fats, every day. You can add flax oil to salad dressings or smoothies, or take it in capsule form—although you'll need to take lots of capsules to get the equivalent of a tablespoon. Refrain from cooking or frying with flax oil, because heat not only destroys its benefits, but could make it detrimental to your health.

2. **Hemp.** Adding hemp seeds to your diet can promote your health and sexual well-being in many ways. Not only are they rich in beneficial omega-3 fats, they're also high in gamma-linolenic acid (GLA). Studies show that GLA reduces inflammation, and can help treat premenstrual syndrome, menopausal hot flashes, osteoporosis, arthritis, heart disease, and other conditions. In addition, hemp seeds are high in vitamins and minerals, and contain all of the essential amino acids. You can find these seeds in many food products, such as hemp milk, hemp oil, hemp flour, and hemp protein powder.

3. **Chia seeds.** An ancient grain from Mexico, chia seeds can pack a lot of extra nutritional power into your Great Sex Diet. They consist of 44 percent carbohydrates—38 percent of which is fiber—31 percent fats, and 16 percent proteins, as well as some antioxidants. Because of their high fiber content, chia seeds support good elimination, and help stabilize your blood sugar, which is advantageous for your sexual energy. Since most of their fats are omega-3 fats, they can be a valuable asset for reducing your risk of heart disease and helping you control cholesterol. You can mix chia seeds into smoothies and soups, or add them to recipes that call for thickeners.

4. **Pumpkin seeds.** An amazing food, pumpkin seeds offer you a diversity of potential health and libido-supportive benefits through their high omega-3 fat content. They can also improve your immunity, decrease your cholesterol, and promote your bone strength. They may also have anti-inflammatory effects that could ease symptoms of arthritis; researchers have found pumpkin-seed oil to be as effective as a well-known anti-inflammatory drug. Pumpkin seeds contain L-tryptophan, a precursor to serotonin, an important neurotransmitter that can affect your sexual health. They also contain an abundance of alpha-linolenic acid, an essential fat that may have benefits for your breast tissue, including potentially helping to prevent breast cancer. Pumpkin seeds are a great addition to your salads, trail mixes, and cereals, and give you a delicious alternative to cow's milk. You may be surprised to discover that the dark green seeds (one cup), blended with just water (five cups), yield a milky-white drink. (Strain, add a dash of vanilla extract, and a touch of stevia to taste.)

5. **Coconut oil.** You might not expect coconut oil to be nominated as a super-libido food. For years, it was mistakenly assumed to be an unsafe saturated fat, but now we know it's a heart-healthy, "friendly" saturated fat with numerous health and immune benefits. The *Journal of Nutrition* has reported that it can help lower your risk of heart disease, and according to the research journal *Obesity,* it may help reduce upper-body fat, prevent obesity, and stimulate weight loss. Heart health supports good circulation, which in turn gives you better overall vitality, including sexual well-being. (Good circulation can be especially beneficial for men's sexual health, and as you'll see later in this book, can help prevent erectile dysfunction.)

6. **Pomegranates.** Modern research confirms that pomegranates, long revered by traditional cultures for their medicinal and sex-promoting properties, contain antioxidants and other compounds that have many health benefits. You've probably seen pomegranate juice promoted as an elixir for men's health concerns, but it offers you plenty of potential benefits, too: supporting your cardiovascular system, improving blood flow to your heart, reducing your blood pressure, increasing your circulation, and

potentially reversing heart disease by inhibiting plaque buildup in your arteries. All of these health gains can enhance female as well as male sexuality.

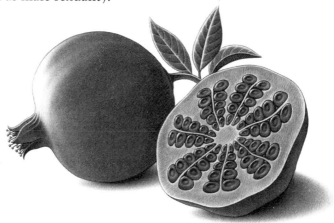

7. **Blueberry juice.** Among the most health-conducive of fruits, loaded with antioxidants, blueberries support the walls of your blood vessels and help protect your brain from oxidative stress. Their protective compounds include anthocyanins (which help protect you from free-radical damage), pterostilbene (an agent that lowers cholesterol and also has anticancer properties), and D-mannose, which can help prevent urinary tract infections. (As you'll see, urinary tract infections have the potential to be a major libido-breaker.) Keep fresh blueberry juice on hand, and enhance your Great Sex Diet by adding a splash of "purple power" to your daily smoothies.

8. **Acai juice.** Another mouthwatering super-juice to jazz up your sex-supportive diet, acai juice can ultimately reinforce your sexuality by boosting your general health. Acai juice is made from berries that have been used for healing purposes by the tribes of the Amazon for centuries. In addition to high levels of anthocyanins that fight free radicals, acai berries contain the health-protective antioxidants vitamin E and vitamin C, plant sterols, and fatty acids, which can all have beneficial effects on your cholesterol levels. Studies have found that acai berries are rich in polyphenols—phytochemicals that also have antioxidant properties and anticancer benefits. Research suggests that acai berries may

help decrease the risk of diabetes and degenerative diseases like arthritis as well, and that extracts of acai berries may be useful in regulating blood pressure and treating cardiovascular disease. Other potential effects include elevating immunity, lowering cholesterol, and slowing the aging process.

9. **Mangosteen juice.** Yet another succulent exotic beverage, mangosteen juice promotes sexual well-being for much the same reason that acai does; mangosteen is rife with health-boosting nutrients. Studies have found that mangosteen fruit contains polysaccharides—carbohydrates that can stimulate immune cells to destroy bacteria—and xanthones (a type of antioxidant) that may help fight cancer. Research also shows that mangosteen has anti-inflammatory effects, and may be useful for treating allergic conditions. Mangosteen juice has a distinct taste that can be described as a combination of pear and strawberry. (Despite its name, mangosteen isn't a member of the mango family.) One caveat regarding its health benefits: most research has been done on the rind of the fruit, and juices may not contain all of the rind's medicinal compounds.

10. **Cruciferous vegetables.** You can fortify your Great Sex Diet every day with the cruciferous family of vegetables, which includes broccoli, cabbage, cauliflower, kale, brussels sprouts, turnip greens, bok choy, radishes, watercress, mustard greens, and collard greens. There's an enormous amount of research on their ability to help your body create friendly forms of estrogen—one of your libido-supportive hormones—and on the anticancer effects of compounds in cruciferous vegetables. Broccoli sprouts, an especially potent member of the cruciferous clan, may contain up to 50 times the concentration of cancer-fighting compounds found in mature broccoli plants.

11. **Green tea.** A much healthier alternative to coffee, green tea (preferably noncaffeinated) may enhance your overall health and support your sexuality by helping prevent cancer and treat human papillomavirus (HPV). The polyphenols in green tea have antioxidant, anti-inflammatory, and anticancer properties, and may help with weight loss as well. Studies have found that green-tea consumption is linked with reduced risk of ovarian cancer and

that survival rates for this form of cancer are higher in women who drink at least one cup daily. Research also shows that green tea may help lower the risk of breast cancer and reduce the growth of a particularly aggressive type of breast-cancer cells. And green-tea extracts have been found to cause improvements in women with HPV-infected cervical lesions, a precursor to cervical cancer, and may also benefit women with vulvar warts.

12. **Shiitake mushrooms.** Long used medicinally in China, shiitake mushrooms make a wonderful, earthy addition to your Great Sex Diet. They provide you with powerful immunity-building glyconutrients—compounds found to improve the ability of immune cells to fight off infections. Shiitake mushrooms not only enhance your resistance to colds and flus, but studies suggest they can also decrease the duration of illnesses. Because of their unique effects on your immunity, shiitakes can play a role in enabling you to manifest peak health and sexual well-being. In addition, research has shown that shiitakes can lower high blood pressure, high cholesterol, and high triglycerides, so you may benefit from consuming them if you have cardiovascular disease (which can hinder healthy sexual functioning).

Sex-Enhancing Exercise

Like your diet, exercise is a part of your life that's completely within your control and can profoundly change your health. We call exercise "sex-enhancing" because it's one of the most important ways you can boost your sexuality with your lifestyle. Let's take a closer look at the sex-enhancing potential of exercise:

— **Exercise is therapy that transforms your entire body.** Your body was made to move; the effects of insufficient exercise, which may include heart disease, arthritis, obesity, and depression, can directly interfere with sexual health. Physical activity can enhance your sexuality by increasing your oxygen intake, strengthening your heart, moving your lymphatic fluids through your body, helping eliminate toxins from your tissues, elevating your vitality, helping you lose weight, and making you look better. By improving the function of every cell in your body, exercise also promotes the healthy functioning of your sexual organs. Ultimately, all exercise is "sexercise."

— **You can specifically enhance your libido with exercise.** Research suggests that women who exercise regularly have increased blood flow to all parts of their bodies, including their pelvic regions, which can improve sexual responsiveness and performance. Exercise can also enhance your libido by decreasing your stress-hormone levels; as you know, stress is a libido-buster.

— **Exercise can increase your energy, which includes your sexual energy.** You can dispel the old notion that exercise always "uses up" your energy or tires you out. To the contrary, by increasing your total number of mitochondria—the energy-producing "engines" in your muscle cells—exercise can boost the amount of energy you have in your body. And improving your overall energy means improving your sexual energy.

— **You can bring more joy into your life, including your sex life, with exercise.** By affecting your neurotransmitters—brain chemicals such as serotonin—exercise can stimulate your brain circuitry into "feel-good" states and alter your moods. Research shows, for example, that women who work out regularly have more confidence in their bodies. A high happiness quotient helps keep you receptive to all the joys of life, including the joys of sex.

Sex Can Make You Skinnier

Like any physical activity, sex can help you lose weight and may even help lower your cholesterol level. You probably burn about 200 calories in 30 minutes of lovemaking, although estimates vary depending on what kinds of sexual activities you engage in. While sex burns some calories, the real reason it can help you lose weight may be that it releases brain chemicals that make you happier, which in turn means you're apt to make healthier choices that tap into your potential to manifest your ideal body size.

Exercise, Motivation, Self-Esteem, and Sex: Rediscovering the Connections

Although your body naturally needs and craves the medicine of exercise, your mind may make excuses—your job, children, other responsibilities, or even your personality or body type—to avoid it. For some women, the mind has a way of coming up with reasons to let the body stay sedentary, even at the risk of poor health, reduced sexual energy, or loss of bodily functions. But knowing all the benefits that exercise has for your health and sexuality can help put your body in motion. Let's look at how you can get your mind more in touch with your natural motivation for motion, and move yourself to move.

When you exercise, you're doing more than simply getting your body in shape and moving your limbs; you're also shaping your mind and moving your emotions. You can think of exercise as *meaningful* movement. In a sense, all exercise is dance: it allows you to celebrate your physical nature in ways that can give you great joy, and you can experience powerful surges of self-confidence when you feel what it's like to manifest potential you might not have known you had. If you've ever learned a dance routine, you may not remember how hesitant you felt when you took your first steps, but you'll probably never forget how confident you felt when you mastered the moves—and still feel whenever you perform them.

No matter how physically inactive you were in the past, or whether you're naturally athletic, discovering new ways of moving can transform your sense of self. Experiencing your body in novel ways can help create new neural tracks in your brain, actually changing how your mental functions work on a daily basis. And the boost in self-esteem you experience from new forms of exercise can enhance your capacity for great sex. When you feel more confident on the dance floor, on the soccer field, or in whatever exercise you choose, your confidence carries over into every other physical activity you engage in—and sex, of course, is no exception.

There's also a lot to be said for the pleasure you can experience by reaching measurable goals and outperforming your personal best. If you swim more laps, walk more miles, or lift more weight than you once thought yourself capable of, it also lifts your spirit and changes your sense of yourself. And while exercise is changing your mind, it's changing your body as well, giving you the added satisfaction of seeing it become fitter.

If you've been physically inactive, and you find the idea of exercise unappealing, it's time to find a form of movement that lets you rediscover the joys of experiencing your body in new ways. Meaningful movement is one of your direct routes to becoming a healthier, happier person, more connected with your body, and more in tune with your sexual energy. And once you're on the move, it's that much easier to keep up your momentum. The more you exercise, the more likely you are to continue to do so. Make it your way of life, and it becomes *you*. The benefits for your health and your sexuality will multiply manyfold; it's the "gift that keeps moving."

Balancing Your Sexuality with Yin and Yang Exercises

Balance is the key when it comes to exercise and your libido; for example, you want to get the benefits of both aerobic exercise and resistance exercise like weight lifting (at least 20 minutes of each, three to four times a week). We can also use the principles of Chinese medicine to create balance by thinking about different types of exercise as either yin or yang. *Yin* exercises are gentler and may involve concentrated focus or "centering" techniques; examples include some forms of yoga and stretching. When you feel stressed, yin exercise can be especially effective in shifting your energy into a calm, relaxed state—from a sympathetic-nervous-system response to a parasympathetic response. *Yang* exercises typically push your body more intensely; examples include mountain climbing with a heavy pack, or running.

Many exercises can be either yin or yang, depending on your approach. Swimming, for instance, can be a mellow yin activity in placid water, or a vigorous yang exercise in rough water. Yoga can likewise be yin or yang; if you take a restorative hatha yoga class, and you hold supported positions while breathing deeply, you're doing a yin form of exercise. On the other hand, if you practice

Bikram yoga for 90 minutes in a heated room, you're practicing a yang form of yoga.

You can support your entire body, reinforce your chi, and help optimize the health of your libido by creating a balance of yin and yang exercises in your life. Too much yin exercise, without enough yang exercise to balance it, can lead to stagnation, low energy, and diminished libido. Excessive yang exercise, without sufficient yin exercise to offset it, can burn out your energy and disrupt your hormonal balance. Energy and balanced hormones are both essential for keeping your sex drive healthy.

You can use the following list of yin and yang exercises as a general guide for creating balance in your life. Each exercise is categorized on the basis of how it's typically experienced by the average person. But again, you can make many activities either yin or yang, depending on the degree of intensity you bring to them.

Yin Exercises	Yang Exercises
Gentle hatha yoga	Bikram or Ashtanga yoga
Light weight lifting	Heavy weight lifting
Walking	Running
Gentle stationary bicycling	Mountain biking
Day hiking without a pack	Mountain climbing
Low-impact aerobics	High-impact aerobics
Slow hula dance	Tahitian dance
Aikido	Kickboxing
Swimming in a lake or pool	Ocean swimming
Low-intensity cross-country skiing	Downhill skiing
Slow ballroom dancing	Fast dancing
Tai chi	Karate
Surfing in small waves	Surfing in big waves
Badminton	Tennis
Canoeing in a slow-moving river	Ocean kayaking

Exercise and Your Pelvis: The Libido Link

Your pelvis is your center of gravity, and it's central to your sexuality. In Chinese medicine, your pelvis is a powerful part of your anatomy—the pivotal area through which all your chi flows from meridians throughout your body. Yet many women feel "blocked," physically or psychologically, from this part of their bodies. They may have freedom of movement and normal sensation in other areas, but because of chronic pelvic pain, sexual issues, or past trauma—or perhaps as a result of growing up in an environment that didn't encourage healthy awareness of their bodies and their sexuality—they remain unconscious of the full range of pelvic sensation they're capable of.

In order to have healthy sex, you need to be comfortable with your body and intimately familiar with your pelvis and sexual organs. One of the best ways to physically and psychologically "reconnect" with your pelvis is through exercises and activities that strengthen and relax your pelvic muscles. This allows you to become more aware of your entire pelvic region and more familiar with sensations in those muscles. It can help you release tensions you may be unconsciously holding in your pelvis, and it may help you discover muscles that you don't know you have. By incorporating the following forms of exercise and movement into your life, you can improve the health of your entire body and your pelvis in particular:

— **Dance.** When the energy of music fills your being and moves your body, no form of exercise is more joyful. And by celebrating your body with dance, you can do more than enhance your health and get in touch with your pelvis; you can dance your way to better sex.

Dance has been practiced by women all over the world since the beginnings of recorded history. In myriad forms of cultural expression, from African dance to the tango, it often involves powerful pelvic muscle movements that can help you maintain core muscle conditioning, increase your pelvic strength, and tone muscles that contract around your vagina.

With so many forms of dance, you can choose whatever fits your personality. One of the best for enhancing your pelvic health is belly dancing. By some accounts, it was taught to young women in ancient Arab tribes for strengthening their pelvic muscles in preparation for childbirth, as well as to ease its effects (although it appears to have originated as entertainment or for erotic purposes). Belly dancing not only tones and strengthens your pelvic muscles, it can also enhance your libido, build your "mind-hip coordination," develop and flatten your stomach muscles, increase circulation throughout your pelvic region, give you a cardiovascular workout, improve your posture, and help prevent osteoporosis.

Another form of dance particularly good for your pelvic health is hula. The graceful, swaying hip motions of Hawaiian hula can increase your pelvic strength and coordination, maintain your pelvic-muscle vitality, and bring chi to your pelvic region. An added attraction is that you can do hula at any age; some of Hawaii's most proficient hula dancers are older women.

You don't need a traditional dance form to enjoy the benefits of this activity. Anytime you feel creative, you can invent your own form of dance right at home: turn on your favorite music, let yourself go, and dance to enhance!

— **Pilates.** When you join the ranks of the Pilates bodies, you're usually instructed, even before you begin the exercises, to tighten your core by contracting the muscles of your lower abdomen and pelvis while pulling up on your pelvic-floor muscles, as if doing a Kegel. (We'll explore Kegel exercises in detail later in this book.) Pilates can be a powerful way of strengthening your core, increasing awareness of your pelvic muscles, and enhancing muscles that contract your vagina during sex.

— **Yoga.** With yoga, you can change your body, including your core, from the inside out. Iyengar yoga, in particular, allows you to increase the flexibility in your hips, buttocks, abdomen, and pelvis. It also enables you to strengthen and tone the muscles of your pelvic region. And while you're expanding your flexibility, it can help you increase your awareness of your posture and lower abdomen.

Your Great Sex Detox

What does throwing out your Teflon pans have to do with having great sex? As you'll discover in the pages ahead, there may be many items in your immediate environment that are compromising your health and affecting your sexual energy. Knowing which to eliminate is part of cleansing your body and enhancing your libido-building lifestyle—which is why we call the cleanse outlined in this section the Great Sex Detox.

If your body is in a toxic state, you don't feel especially sexy or attractive. You probably feel tired, achy, and as if you have a hangover most of the time. Imagine what your life would be like if you didn't take the garbage out of your living space for months, or years; that's analogous to what happens to your tissues if you don't detoxify your body. It's no wonder if you feel literally "down in the dumps."

By eliminating toxins accumulated in your body, the Great Sex Detox can recharge your energy, boost your libido, promote clearer thinking, support your brain health, elevate your moods by increasing the synthesis of "happy" neurotransmitters, improve your digestive health, help your liver work better, balance and strengthen your chi, help you lose weight if you need to, and more. It can make you feel more alive, and sexier, than you may have felt in years. After following this unique cleanse, many of my patients report having more energy and improved sleep, and say they feel "born again." It's about cleansing your body of impurities on a cellular level, as well as creating long-lasting behavioral changes and giving you a sense of empowerment.

The Great Sex Detox can also improve your hormone metabolism by boosting your intake of cruciferous vegetables, which contain compounds that help break down estrogen in your body. As you'll discover in a subsequent chapter, you have better hormonal health, and better overall health—as well as potentially better sex—when your body does a good job of breaking down estrogen into its "friendly," rather than "unfriendly," forms. (There are many types of estrogen; you want to convert estrogens into weaker, friendlier forms—not unfriendly ones.) The friendly forms of estrogen help moisten your skin, hydrate your vagina, create pleasant moods, and support the functioning of your memory;

the unfriendly ones may contribute to ovarian cysts, fibroids, cystic breasts, breast cancer, and a host of other problems.

The Great Sex Detox is easy to implement, and you can continue with all of your normal, everyday activities—your job, exercise, taking care of the kids, walking the dog, and so on—while you're doing it. It's a relatively gentle cleanse, unlike some aggressive detox plans that can be physically draining and interrupt your lifestyle. You should feel good while you're doing the Great Sex Detox, and since you'll be releasing toxins that may have been stored in your body for many years, you can expect to feel increasingly better as your cleanse progresses.

While you're doing the Great Sex Detox, you can continue taking prescription medications—for example, if you're on high-blood-pressure medication—but check with your doctor first. Abstain from all alcohol, recreational drugs, and smoking. It's best to eat only organic foods, and important to avoid all junk foods, refined sugars, fried foods, and processed food products.

Getting Started:
Remove the Obstacles to Health and Pleasure

Some people have the misguided notion that a cleanse involves only your body. But to be effective, it should also involve your surroundings, because some of the pollutants you want to eradicate from your tissues may come from common consumer products you're exposed to right in your own home. Every day, you may be running a gauntlet of chemical assailants with potentially serious consequences for your health and sexuality. If you don't remove them *before* you begin cleansing your body, your cleanse may have limited benefits—like bailing out a leaky boat without plugging the holes.

This is why it's essential to launch the Great Sex Detox by finding natural alternatives for as many items as you can that may release toxic chemicals in or around your household—including your cleaning products, cookware, personal-care products, food-storage containers, and more.

35

— The **cleaning products** stocked in many homes are a case of chemical overkill, needlessly laced with powerful toxic chemicals. Numerous household cleaning agents include cancer-causing compounds, neurotoxins, chemicals associated with decidedly unsexy symptoms, and ingredients linked to birth defects. There's a plethora of safe, natural alternatives you can use to keep your home clean—arguably much *cleaner* than if you use toxic pollutants—and you probably already have a number of healthy options on hand. Vinegar, baking soda, lemon juice, castile soap, borax, and salt can be used in various combinations, with a little practice, to meet all your cleaning needs. You can find suggestions for cleaning your home safely by browsing the website of the Environmental Working Group (EWG), and nontoxic cleaning agents are available at many health-food stores.

— Next, let's take a look at your **cookware**, and those Teflon pans. If you use nonstick pans to cook with, you may be exposing yourself to potential health risks that can seriously subvert your sexual energy. Sure, they're convenient, but at what awful price? According to a 2006 news release from the EWG, a panel of experts confirmed that a toxic chemical used in nonstick pans can cause cancer, and may be associated with birth defects and other health risks. The chemical, which doesn't break down in the environment, ends up in your bloodstream when you use these pans. Healthy alternatives to nonstick pans include stainless-steel and cast-iron cookware.

— Another area of concern, your **personal-care products**, includes everything from your shampoo, deodorant, and toothpaste to your makeup and nail polish. Many commonly used items contain ingredients that are neither health-supportive nor libido-friendly. Some contain phthalates and other potentially harmful synthetic chemicals, including ingredients that could be potentially cancer initiating. Safe, healthy alternatives to chemically laden personal-care items abound at your local health-food stores and online. For information on chemicals in your cosmetics, visit the EWG's Skin Deep website at: **www.cosmeticsdatabase.com**.

— And what about your **food-storage containers**? You may not be aware that the chemical *bisphenol A,* or BPA, found in many plastics and commonly used in containers, can be released into foods and beverages, especially with temperature elevations. BPA can compromise your health and sexuality in multiple ways: it has estrogen-mimicking effects; potentially causes hormone disruptions in women and men; and may contribute to infertility, breast cancer, and early puberty in girls. Furthermore, exposure to BPA during pregnancy could negatively affect the fetus. To decrease your exposure, replace plastic food containers with glassware, and avoid canned foods if the cans have epoxy liners—a frequent source of BPA. If you drink from plastic water bottles, switch to glass or stainless steel.

In addition, you need to examine every other aspect of your home environment and daily routines, and ask yourself where you may be coming into contact with chemicals that could undermine your health and libido. For example, your sunscreens, laundry detergents, dry-cleaning services, pest-control treatments, and yard products like weed killers and fertilizers can all be sources of toxins and unhealthy, antisexual synthetic compounds. Another concern may be automatic-dishwasher soaps that include ingredients you wouldn't want to ingest, even in minuscule amounts— and those "spot removers" for dishes that contain known skin irritants. And don't forget about your medicines and health-care products, which all too often can be sources of questionable chemicals. (See sidebar, and if you use birth control, see Appendix H.) Remember that when it comes to your health and libido, less is more; if in doubt, leave it out. Your vigilance in rooting out hidden health foes and sex saboteurs, and eliminating them from your personal surroundings, will contribute to the success of your Great Sex Detox.

To learn more about the potential health effects of many chemicals found in products you may be using in or around your living area, visit: **www.ewg.org**.

Can Your Medicines Be Unhealthy?

If you comb your medicine cabinet, reading the fine print on products like cough medicines, nasal decongestants, antihistamines, and diet aids, you may be surprised by what you find. Many products contain synthetic additives, fillers, or colorings, some of which may even be listed by the EWG as hazardous to one degree or another. Eliminate anything you can do without; with a little research, you can find healthy natural remedies to replace a wide variety of health-care products. If you need assistance, consult a licensed naturopathic physician. (See Appendix B to find one.)

As you research your alternatives, keep in mind that natural remedies—including some that have been used for centuries—have a big disadvantage in the world of modern pharmaceutical medicine: large drug companies seeking to patent and market nonnatural products typically conduct numerous studies in an effort to prove their effectiveness, while natural substances, which can't legally be patented, often get ignored. As a result, the number of studies on natural remedies may seem small by comparison—prompting misleading claims that there's relatively little evidence to prove their effectiveness. With a few sound bites, public-relations firms hired by pharmaceutical giants can discredit natural remedies that, in some cases, have stood the test of time, were held in trust by your ancestors, and have been passed down to you over many generations.

Your Great Sex Detox Dietary Cleanse

Once you've cleaned up as many health- and sex-negating chemicals as you can in your home environment, you're ready to begin cleansing your body. The dietary cleanse that is part of the Great Sex Detox is a three-week plan, and to optimize its benefits, you should adhere to all of the recommendations outlined in the remainder of the chapter for the full 21 days. After you've completed this dietary cleanse, its benefits—along with all the others you experience from the Great Sex Detox—will be ongoing. The dietary cleanse is essentially a way to jump-start your body's detoxification systems; once they're revved up, they'll continue working optimally if you keep eating well and exercising. (And after the cleanse, you can continue to include "magic" smoothies, as described in this section, in your diet indefinitely.)

The Great Sex Detox dietary cleanse is specifically designed to enhance your overall health and sexual well-being by ridding toxic pollutants from your tissues, and it has many other benefits as well. It's hypoallergenic (it protects you from most common allergens), and provides you with lots of healthy fiber from nutritious vegetables, salads, and smoothies. You may notice that all of this fiber improves the regularity of your bowel movements. This can benefit your hormonal health, which in turn can further enhance your overall energy, vitality, and libido.

Here's an overview of your dietary cleanse, and what you need to do in order to get the best results from it:

— **Limit your grain intake to five foods.** Consume rice, quinoa, amaranth, tapioca, and buckwheat. These grains are free of gluten, a common allergen, and abstaining from other grains relieves you of potential allergic symptoms that can hinder your health and libido. You can eat whatever quantity of grains you want, as long as you restrict the grain portion of your diet to these five.

— **Eat lots of vegetables.** On as many days as possible, enjoy a large salad, including several different-colored vegetables—for example, carrots, cucumbers, tomatoes, peppers, and lettuce. Also eat, on as many days as you can, a half cup of broccoli sprouts and at least two cruciferous vegetables (identified earlier in this chapter as one of your super-libido foods).

— **Consume oils that support your health and sexuality.** These include flax, olive, and fish oil; also eat nuts and seeds that contain beneficial oils, as well as avocados. If you cook with oil, use olive, canola, macadamia-nut, or coconut oil.

— **Avoid dairy and egg products.** Cows and other animals remove toxins from their bodies, in part, by excreting milk, so when you consume dairy products, you may expose yourself to increased toxins that can hamper your health and libido. Dairy products can also be particularly high in allergens, and many people have low-grade allergies to dairy or eggs without realizing it. Eliminating them during your dietary cleanse gives your digestive system a break from potentially unhealthful, unsexy symptoms.

— **Limit your protein sources to certain healthy foods.** Meet your protein needs by consuming only organic skinless lean chicken or turkey; wild salmon (avoid farm-raised); kidney, garbanzo, navy, or pinto beans (exclude soybeans, another common allergen); and lentils, peas, seeds, and nuts (but avoid peanuts and peanut butter).

— **Eat until you're full, but don't overeat.** You shouldn't be excessively hungry, or overly full, during your dietary cleanse. To keep your blood sugar even—which, as you've seen, helps regulate your energy and libido—eat three meals a day, and two daily snacks if you like.

— **Enjoy "magic" smoothies daily.** Your magic smoothie, which includes some of your super-libido foods, consists of fruits, vegetables, and other ingredients. Blend as many of the following as you can in each of your smoothies. Since chia seeds can thicken your smoothie, you might want to add extra water, or blend them in last.

MAGIC SMOOTHIE RECIPE
2 Tbsp. rice-based protein powder (see Appendix C)
1 tsp. cinnamon
1 cup parsley, spinach, or kale
1 small carrot (approx. 4 inches in length)
2 inches cucumber
1 or 2 inches zucchini, or similar amount of broccoli
½ apple
½ cup blueberries
1 Tbsp. pumpkin seeds
1 Tbsp. chia seeds
1½ cups water

— **Minimize your fruit intake.** Limit your daily fruit consumption to two cups, or two pieces, of low-glycemic fruit, which includes apples, pears, cherries, apricots, plums, peaches, oranges, blueberries, blackberries, raspberries, and strawberries. As pointed out earlier in this chapter, some fruits are super-libido foods, but at the same time excessive intake of fruit sugar can disrupt your blood-sugar level, which is detrimental to your health and sexual energy.

— **Add lemon juice to your water.** Lemon juice supports your dietary cleanse by promoting the health of your liver, your body's master cleansing organ. Squeeze the juice from a quarter of a medium-size lemon into 12 ounces of water, and sip during the day. Doing this two to three times daily will also help ensure that you're getting plenty of water, which supports all your body's tissues, including your sex organs. (If you have a history of heartburn, you may need to refrain from using lemon in your water.)

If you faithfully follow these dietary guidelines during your three-week dietary cleanse, you're likely to be extremely pleased with the results and the potential rejuvenating effects on your health and sexual energy. For a day-by-day outline of the meal and supplement portions of your cleanse, see Appendix D.

Supplements to Enhance Your
Great Sex Detox Dietary Cleanse

While you're cleansing your body with your dietary choices, you need to take the right supplements to maximize your ability to eliminate undesirable elements that can encumber your health and libido. The supplements you'll take each day during your 21-day dietary cleanse (some of these can be found in Appendix C), along with an overview of how they can help detoxify your tissues and give you other benefits, are listed here. You can discontinue taking some of these supplements after the 21 days, but you should continue with the antioxidant formula, multivitamin, and flax oil indefinitely.

— **Liver lipotropic formula.** This formula consists of herbs and nutrients to help your liver more effectively break down toxins, which assists in their removal from your body. Take two capsules of liver lipotropic formula (see Appendix C) twice daily during your 21-day cleanse. You probably won't want to add this to your smoothies because of the taste.

— **Chlorella.** A type of green algae that emerged on Earth billions of years ago, chlorella is a rich source of chlorophyll consisting of 50 percent proteins, 23 percent carbohydrates, 12 percent healthy fats, the antioxidant beta-carotene, and numerous vitamins and minerals. Chlorella is important in your dietary cleanse because it can assist in the removal of unhealthy, unsexy toxins from your body—including environmental chemicals such as dioxin and heavy metals like mercury and lead—and render some harmless. It can also improve your digestion, support the health of your intestinal environment, enhance the growth of friendly bacteria in your digestive system, and boost your immunity. As an added bonus, it helps freshen your breath. Take two 300 mg chlorella pills (see Appendix C) twice daily with water, or add them to your smoothies, during your 21-day cleanse.

— **Antioxidant formula.** Make sure that you keep taking your antioxidants, as outlined previously in this chapter, during your dietary cleanse. This aids your liver in breaking down toxins so it is easier for your body to eliminate them. To use the antioxidant formula in Appendix C, take two capsules daily during your cleanse. (You can blend them into your smoothies if you like.)

— **Multivitamin.** Continuing to take your daily multivitamin, as described earlier in this chapter, is an important part of your dietary cleanse because it gives your body the nutrition it needs to help eliminate toxins that can obstruct your health and libido. There's no telling how many toxic chemicals and pollutants you've been exposed to, so you want to be sure you're getting this baseline of nutrients. If you opt to take the multivitamin in Appendix C, consume two tablets twice daily with food during your cleanse. (You can also blend these into your smoothies.)

—**Flax oil.** As you've discovered, flax is a super-libido food rich in friendly omega-3 fats, and flax oil gives you many health benefits. It helps with your dietary cleanse by promoting your body's ability to remove toxins from every cell in your body. Be sure that you're getting one tablespoon of flax oil every day of your cleanse. You can mix it into salad dressings, pour it over vegetable dishes, or add it to smoothies. You can also take it in capsule form, if you don't mind taking enough capsules to equal a tablespoon.

— **Friendly bacteria.** Friendly bacteria support your dietary cleanse and promote your health and sexuality in many ways. These supplements encourage the growth of other beneficial bacteria in your intestinal walls, help protect your intestines from pathogens like parasites, help break down compounds that could initiate cancer, and assist your body in making nutrients. Take at least a billion organisms of the friendly bacteria in Appendix C once a day with water, or added to your smoothies, during your cleanse.

— **Antibug herbs.** You may have any number of microscopic "bugs," including hidden parasites, bacteria, and yeast, inhabiting your intestines, especially if you experience chronic gas and bloating. These bugs can have many effects that thwart your health and limit your sexual energy, and their number is related to the overall toxicity of your body; they essentially exert harmful effects and reduce your body's effectiveness in dealing with your cumulative toxic burden. Antibug herbs support your dietary cleanse by rearranging your gut flora to give you a healthier intestinal wall. They also strengthen your immune system, help liberate your libido from undesirable symptoms, and can assist in lowering blood pressure and cholesterol.

For the duration of your dietary cleanse, take either of the following (available at many health-food stores) three times a day with food: one 900 mg garlic pill containing 5,000 mcg of allicin, or one berberine pill (a standardized extract containing 200 mg per pill). Berberine shouldn't be used during pregnancy or lactation.

It's important to adhere to these guidelines regarding your supplement regimen during your three-week dietary cleanse. (Again, refer to the outline in Appendix D for a day-by-day breakdown of the meal and supplement portions of your cleanse.)

Other Tools for Enhancing Your Dietary Cleanse

While you're eliminating toxins from your tissues with your dietary cleanse, there are a few additional steps that can help rid your body of unwanted contaminants. The following measures serve as catalysts by speeding up your body's ability to shed toxins, and at the same time they increase the energy- and libido-building benefits of your dietary cleanse. After completing your 21-day cleanse, you can continue using these techniques indefinitely to optimize your potential to detoxify.

— **Great sweats, naturally.** Perspiration can be a key factor in the success of your dietary cleanse, because it's one of your body's most efficient ways of purging toxins. You can work up a healthy sweat with any kind of aerobic exercise, but one of the best ways to send your toxins packing is with a dry sauna. When you use a low-heat sauna for 60 to 90 minutes, your body begins to mobilize toxins out of your fat cells, into your blood, and out through your sweat.

Make a point to sweat out your toxins at least twice a week during your dietary cleanse. If your local health club or spa has a dry sauna that allows you to adjust the heat, you can find the temperature that suits you best. (The ideal for many people is about 105 degrees Fahrenheit, but it can vary from one person to the next.) Another great option is Bikram yoga, an advanced form of yoga done in a room heated to about 105 degrees. Keep your tissues hydrated by drinking plenty of fluids before and after a sauna or Bikram yoga class.

— **Dry-skin brushing.** You can further facilitate detoxification by skin brushing, because your skin accumulates toxins your body is trying to eliminate through your pores. You need to keep your skin—your body's largest sex organ—as clean and healthy as possible. Because of its extensive surface area, you may be harboring a substantial residue of toxins and dead cells on your outer surface. Perhaps you've done everything right with your dietary cleanse, released toxins out of your pores, and have all but gotten rid of them—yet they still cling to the outside of your body. All you have to do is brush them off and they're gone forever.

Skin brushing not only clears toxins and dead skin from the surface of your body, it also stimulates your blood and lymph vessels—both of which remove toxins and other debris from your cells. Do skin brushing at least once every day during your dietary cleanse; you may be surprised by how revitalized you feel after such a simple technique. With a soft scrub brush, use gentle, firm strokes to cover as much of your body as possible, always brushing toward your chest. (To most effectively enhance detoxification, it's best to encourage the circulation of your lymphatic fluids in the direction of your heart.) Brush from your hands toward your shoulders, and from your feet toward your pelvis; upward from your abdomen and lower back toward your heart; and downward from your neck toward your heart. As an alternative to dry-skin brushing, you can use a loofah sponge or exfoliating glove in the shower.

Conclusion: Putting the Great Sex Lifestyle into Action

In this chapter, you've explored three highly significant aspects of your health and sexuality: your diet, exercise habits, and ability to detoxify. You've seen the vast difference that each can make in your overall health and your capacity for sexual pleasure.

We began this chapter by reflecting on the notion that great sex is your birthright, but with an important caveat: you ultimately have to *choose* it. As you move ahead, you can use the tools you've just discovered to make choices that will maximize the effects of everything else you gain from this book—whether it's new exercises, acupressure points, specific aphrodisiacs, or any other way of enhancing your sexuality or health. So let's continue moving forward; the journey has only just begun, and there's much more to discover. . . .

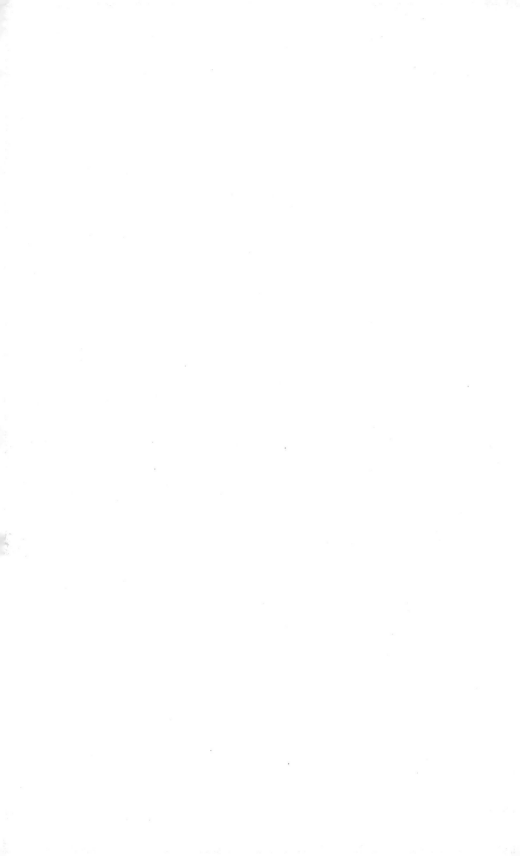

CHAPTER 3

YOUR
SEXUAL
CORE

Creating Optimal Pelvic and Vaginal Health

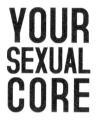

"Electric flesh-arrows . . . traversing the body.
A rainbow of color strikes the eyelids. A foam of music
falls over the ears. It is the gong of the orgasm."

— ANAÏS NIN, *DIARY OF ANAÏS NIN*

47

As we pointed out in Chapter 1, your body is perfectly designed for great sex. You have all the right ingredients—nerves, hormones, glands, and other physiological components—to reach the highest states of sexual ecstasy. In this chapter, we'll explore the critical role of your pelvic region, look at what you need to know to intensify sexual pleasure in your genitals and other pelvic organs, and provide you with exercises and various tools for strengthening your pelvis and further enhancing your sexuality. If you experience common challenges that women encounter in this vital area of their bodies—such as vaginal dryness, vaginal or urinary infections, menstrual cramps, or chronic pelvic pain—you'll also discover many effective natural solutions.

Your pelvis allows you to move through the world with balance, stability, and strength. One of the most dynamic areas of your body, it also allows you to make love, achieve orgasm, menstruate, release eggs for potential new life, and develop a fetus. In addition, it supports your bladder and other vital organs, and enables the elimination of wastes so the rest of your body can operate efficiently. Your pelvis not only is your center of gravity, but also the core of your sexuality, the seat of your genitals, and the site of thousands of nerve endings with no other purpose than to give you sensual pleasure.

In Chinese medicine, your pelvis is also seen as central—an energetic hothouse of chi. All the chi in your body flows through your powerful pelvis; you can nourish this area and resolve many pelvic and sexual issues by increasing the circulation of your chi. As you'll discover, this may be especially important if you have what's referred to as "stuck chi" in your pelvic region.

Your body has other erogenous zones, beyond your pelvis and genitalia, that contribute to your sexuality and overall health. But your pelvis is so pivotal, on so many levels, that it merits special focus. Let's begin by exploring the anatomical nature of your pelvic organs and genitals, and the key roles they play in your sexual health and pleasure.

The Intimate Anatomy of Your Pelvis

The framework of your pelvis is composed mainly of the two large hip bones that spread out to support your lower body. Within this structure, an elaborate network of muscles and ligaments works to embrace your internal organs, help hold your body upright, and enhance your sexual functions.

Your pelvic muscles consist of an outer, middle, and inner layer. The outer layer, which lies just beneath your skin, can be imperative for orgasms because it contains parts of your clitoris. (As you'll discover, your clitoris is more voluminous than you may think.) The muscles that form the middle layer are important for your sexuality not only because they surround your vagina, but also because they give additional support to portions of your clitoris—your clitoral bulbs. Your urethra passes through these middle-layer muscles as well, so keeping them strong can help prevent urinary incontinence.

The inner layer of your pelvic muscles, known as your *pelvic diaphragm,* includes your pubococcygeal (PC) muscle, which contracts rhythmically when you have orgasms and can contribute to their intensity. (The PC muscle is actually more than one muscle, but is traditionally referred to in the singular, as we do here.) This muscle is also essential for supporting your genital organs and bladder. It runs from the front to the back of your pelvis (from your pubic bone to your anus), and from one side of your pelvis to the other, creating a large bowl-shaped "hammock" that holds up your pelvic organs. If your PC muscle is well toned, it's tight and supportive; if not, it's loose and saggy, which can result in incontinence. It can also lead to organ prolapse—a condition in which the structures that normally hold up an organ are no longer sufficiently supportive, and it "falls down."

Along with your three layers of pelvic muscles, you have multipurpose pelvic ligaments that support your sexuality by connecting your clitoris to your uterus, allowing you to feel deep uterine pleasure during sex and orgasm. In addition, your pelvic ligaments not only structurally support your uterus, but also move it, along with your cervix, up and out of the way during intercourse.

Your Phenomenal Feminine Organs

49

Your sexual organs, the centerpiece of your pelvis, are a wonder of nature, unique in their elegance, complexity, and capacity to bring you to shivering heights of sensual pleasure and profound feelings of spiritual connection and love. With their ability to expand and contract, respond and recoil, welcome and release, they're delightfully dualistic; partly external and partly internal, both seen and unseen, closely known yet secretive and mysterious. In Chinese medical terms, they're both yang (outward, in the light, "hot," and intense), and yin (inward, dark, cool, and protected). Let's take a closer look at each of your precious sex organs:

— **Your vulva.** The beautiful outer portion of your feminine organs, your soft, velvety vulva suggests the shape of an orchid in bloom. The term *vulva* encompasses your labia majora (the large outer lips along the entrance to your vagina), labia minora (your thinner, inner vaginal lips), vaginal opening, external clitoris, and urethral opening. Your vulva contains thousands of nerve endings, includes glands that allow for vaginal lubrication, and provides a protective covering for your inner structures and organs. Your vulva also includes your mons veneris (Latin for "mountain of Venus"), the soft mound over your pubic bone.

— **Your clitoris.** Perhaps the single clearest anatomical proof that you're meant to enjoy your sexuality, your clitoris has but one purpose: to give you pleasure. (It may be no coincidence that the words *clitoris* and *climax* share a common Indo-European root.) Resting partly on the outside of your body yet nestled inside your protective external labia and hidden beneath its hood, your clitoris contains highly specialized, delicate tissue and between 6,000 and 8,000 touch-sensitive nerve endings—a staggeringly dense concentration compared to other similarly sized parts of your body.

Dictionaries typically define the clitoris as a "small" erectile organ, but you may be surprised and delighted to learn that your clitoris is much larger and more extensive than what you can see externally. Many women believe that the clitoris consists only of the "nub" (the clitoral glans) that protrudes below the pubic bone, along with its cape (the protective clitoral hood, or *prepuce*). In fact, the visible portions of your clitoris are only the beginning.

Your clitoral anatomy also includes the shaft of your clitoris, which is directly under the glans, and the two wing-shaped "legs," or *crura* (*crus* is the singular), of your clitoris. Your crura, which are made of erectile tissue, support your clitoral shaft and curve downward and to the sides for approximately four inches along your pubic arch. In addition, you have two clitoral "bulbs," also known as *vestibular bulbs,* extending downward from your clitoral shaft for three to five inches along both sides of your inner labia and your urethral and vaginal openings. Also made of erectile tissue, your clitoral bulbs become swollen and engorged with blood when you're aroused. (*Erectile tissue* generally refers to spongy tissue that expands and becomes firmer when filled with blood.

The term is so often associated with a man's anatomy that some women are surprised to learn they have erectile tissue, too.)

— **Your perineum.** The area of strong, supportive muscle tissue between your vagina and your anus, your perineum contains your perineal sponge, which becomes engorged with blood and swells up when you're aroused. For some women, the surface of the central perineum is highly sensitive to touch and is a source of pleasure when stroked or gently massaged.

The perineum has special significance in more than one Eastern tradition. In the chakra system of Hinduism, it's the location of the *Muladhara* or root chakra, which is associated with birth, life, safety, sexuality, and your connection with the earth. And in Chinese medicine, the center of your perineum is the site of an important acupressure point called *Conception Vessel 1,* also known as *Hui Yin,* which means "meeting of yin." Your yin (the feminine aspect of your chi, as the Introduction to this book touched on) is concentrated at this point, and pressing on it can strengthen your chi and bring you many health benefits, including enhanced sexual energy.

— **Your vagina.** The flexible, enfolding tunnel of your vagina extends deeply into your body, and elongates when you're sexually aroused. As the threshold to your cervix, uterus, fallopian tubes, and ovaries, it's an especially yin organ—internal, receptive, dark, moist, and resilient. Healthy levels of hormones in your body, particularly estrogen, thicken and "fluff up" the tissues of your vagina, helping maintain their pH levels and support their integrity and elasticity.

Your vagina includes your G-spot (the *Grafenberg spot,* sometimes referred to as the *Goddess spot*), well known for its ability to stimulate mind-blowing orgasms. To find your G-spot, use your index or middle finger to reach one to two inches inside your vagina, in the direction of your clitoris; curl your finger upward, and feel along the center of the anterior (front) of your vaginal wall—as if you're reaching toward the side of your body that your navel is on. (For many women, it's easier to find the G-spot when aroused, for reasons we'll explore in the pages ahead.)

51

— **Your urethral sponge, or G-sponge.** People are often un-aware of the potential role that a woman's urethral sponge—not to be confused with her perineal sponge—can play in sexual plea-sure. Your urethral sponge, the female counterpart of the male prostate gland, is sometimes called the female prostate. Located di-rectly behind your G-spot, it's made up of erectile tissue and para-urethral glands that assist with your sexual response and arousal. The glands in your urethral sponge can produce fluid resembling male prostatic fluid (although more watery), and as you'll discover later in this chapter, when sufficiently aroused, some women ejac-ulate this fluid from their bodies. Because of the close proximity of the urethral sponge to the G-spot, and its notable capacity to enhance arousal, we sometimes refer to it as the *G-sponge.*

— **Your cervix.** The narrow entrance at the top of your va-gina, your cervix helps create lubrication during sex and provides a passageway for sperm on their way to your uterus. Your os (the opening of your cervix) is very yin—tightly contracted, with a width of only a few millimeters—but also has the capacity to be extremely yang. As the gateway that most of us passed through on our journey into the world, it can expand to an astounding ten centimeters during childbirth.

— **Your uterus.** Your cervix opens to your uterus, your inner sanctum—and if you procreate, your baby's first home. Although held in place by ligaments and pelvic muscles, the uterus isn't stat-ic, contrary to what many women think; it can frequently shift position inside your pelvic cavity. During sex it moves upward, away from the internal dance, yet it continues to take part in the performance.

During your menstruating years, your monthly flow keeps you acutely aware of the power and presence of your uterus. Every month, tissue inside your uterus known as the *endometrium,* stim-ulated by your hormones, builds a soft, nourishing bed for the prospect of pregnancy. If you don't become pregnant, you shed and release your endometrial lining as your monthly menstrual flow. If you become pregnant, your uterus expands dramatically; it can grow from a mere two ounces to about two pounds toward the end of pregnancy.

— **Your fallopian tubes.** From the top portion of your uterus, your fallopian tubes extend gracefully upward toward your ovaries. Every month during your ovulating years a ripe egg, newly released from your ovaries, floats in the small, nebulous inner cavity of your pelvis directly above your fallopian tubes. Like a sea anemone collecting microscopic nutrients in the ocean current, fluttering tentacles at the ends of your fallopian tubes reach, embrace, and gently guide the egg down into the central tube toward your uterus. In *Woman: An Intimate Geography,* science writer Natalie Angier describes the fallopian tubes as "exquisite, soft and rosy and slim . . . tipped like a feather duster with a bell of fronds, called fimbriae." If traveling sperm find their way to the egg, it could become fertilized; although millions of sperm may surround it, only one might become interlocked with the future.

— **Your ovaries.** Small but powerful glands, your ovaries do even more than produce thousands of eggs with the potential to create new life; they also release estrogen, progesterone, DHEA, and testosterone. All of these hormones can affect your sexuality, your nervous system, and your brain, with far-reaching consequences in your life. Women who have their ovaries removed and don't take replacement hormones typically report feeling changed in every aspect of their being. In the next chapter, you'll discover the great impact that hormones released by your ovaries can have on the quality of your life.

A Word about Words:
The Power of Naming Your Sexual Parts

For purposes of this book we've used the common, usually Latin-derived terms for sexual organs, such as *vulva, vagina, clitoris,* and *penis.* These terms are perfectly acceptable, but for some they may inadequately reflect the sense that pelvic anatomy is a sacred area of the body. If you grew up in an atmosphere where words describing genitals were considered "dirty" or shameful, such terms may carry less-than-inspiring connotations.

Other cultural traditions sometimes offer refreshing perspectives on naming parts of sexual anatomy. In the Hindu tradition, for instance, a woman's genitals (her vulva as well as her vagina) are referred to as her *yoni,* which in Sanskrit means "abode" or "source."

The yoni is considered a symbol of the goddess Shakti, who represents female creative power, and is sometimes referred to as the sacred space, divine passage, or temple. In ancient China, a woman's pubic hair was sometimes described as her fragrant moss, or her black rose.

In some tantric teachings, a woman's yoni is known as her *jade gate*, *lotus*, or *lotus valley* (fittingly, the English word *valley* derives from the same root as *vulva*). Her clitoris may be referred to as her *pearl*, or *bliss pearl*, and her anus—in stark contrast with that word's connotations—as her *rosebud*. Her partner's sexual parts likewise have names conveying beautiful or empowering images. His penis may be referred to as the *lingam*, which in Hinduism is a symbol of male creative energy and is representative of the god Shiva. Tantric teachings sometimes refer to the penis as a *tool for healing, wand of light, jade stalk, diamond scepter,* or *thunderbolt of wisdom;* his testicles may be called *elixir-filled jewels,* his prostate the *sacred sector,* and his semen the *elixir of life.*

According to these designations, the sexual act can consist of a man's wand of light entering a woman's sacred space, stimulating her bliss pearl, and inducing his jewels to release the elixir of life. What a difference words can make! Imagine living in a culture that consistently honored sexual parts with such names.

The Many-Splendored Pleasures of Your Pelvis

Of all the mysteries your pelvis holds, perhaps most awe-inspiring is its potential for multiple modes of ecstasy. Your sexual organs allow you to experience a magnificent variety of indescribable sensations, and the pathways to orgasm can vary widely from one woman to the next. The pace varies as well; some women ride to the crest of the wave with relative ease, while others need more prolonged coaxing.

Even the psychological approach to orgasm differs broadly among women. For example, some women experience orgasm as a purely physical experience with little or no element of sexual fantasy, while for others orgasm is accompanied by elaborate fantasies and visualizations. And it appears that some women may even be able to climax without any physical stimulation; sex researcher Alfred Kinsey famously found that 2 percent of women were able to reach orgasm entirely through fantasy.

A woman's journey to full arousal also differs considerably from a man's. A man often feels ready for orgasm relatively quickly, but a woman typically needs more extensive foreplay. Her sexual energy warms up at its own natural tempo, moving gradually from the outer edges of her body toward her sexual center before she's ready for full arousal and direct stimulation of her sexual organs. And after climax, a woman doesn't need an extended refractory period, as a man does, before experiencing another orgasm; her body allows her to continue riding the wave with multiple orgasms.

The distinction between the timing of male and female sexual energy can be compared to heating up two differently sized pots of water: A man is like a small pot on a large flame; he heats up quickly, and cools rapidly when the flame subsides. A woman is like a large pot on a small flame; she takes more time to heat up, but stays hot for a longer time.

This difference is reflected in Chinese medicine: as the introduction to this book described, male energy is predominantly yang, hot, and outward; and female energy tends to be yin, cool, and inward. (We'll explore ways of balancing yin and yang sexual energies later in this book.) For many women to reach orgasm, however, they need to be not only in touch with their feminine, yin energy—which helps them feel relaxed and safe, release control, and surrender to sensual touch—but also with the yang energy that can give them fiery passion and intensity.

What Happens When You Become Aroused and Reach Orgasm?

As you become aroused, the blood flow to your pelvis increases, engorging your labia, clitoris, and vagina, and you begin to release vaginal lubrication. The tissues of your vulva become, in a sense, more vital and "robust." In *Women's Anatomy of Arousal*, Sheri Winston points out that with arousal your vulva "blooms open like a fleshy fertile flower." Your clitoris becomes "erect," much like a man's penis does but on a different scale, and as your vagina becomes increasingly engorged with fluids, it also expands, becoming longer and wider. At the same time, your PC muscle, which forms the "hammock" that supports your pelvic organs, tightens.

During arousal, with stimulation of your clitoris, vagina, cervix, breasts, or nipples, your body can begin to release oxytocin—the "love hormone" that, as you discovered in Chapter 1, plays a profound role in your ability to bond with your partner. This release may cause vaginal, cervical, and uterine contractions, heightening your arousal. In an escalating feedback loop, continued arousal and stimulation can in turn promote the release of more oxytocin, which can increasingly intensify your contractions and pleasure.

With orgasm, your brain releases a surge of oxytocin that further enhances bonding and releases endorphins that contribute to your experience of all-encompassing euphoria. As your awareness is flooded with pleasure, areas of your brain momentarily disengage from their normal activities. Orgasm is also accompanied by a dramatic increase in your heart rate, an additional surge of blood flow to your pelvic region, an increase in your vagina's lubrication, and contractions of your pelvic muscles, including intense spasms of your PC muscle at brief intervals. At the same time, many muscles throughout your body contract and quiver. Typically, your vagina and uterus also contract rhythmically, and your clitoris tucks in under its hood.

The changes that naturally take place in your body during orgasm can bring you innumerable health benefits; as we emphasized earlier in this book, not only does great health promote great sex, but great sex promotes great health. Modern research confirms what has been recognized for millennia in Chinese medicine: sex and orgasm are especially good for your health, and women who experience regular orgasms have increased circulation of pelvic chi and greater overall vitality.

Regular orgasms increase your pelvic blood flow, strengthen your pelvic muscles, and stimulate your natural vaginal lubrication (which helps prevent chronic vaginal dryness). According to Barry R. Komisaruk, Carlos Beyer-Flores, and Beverly Whipple in *The Science of Orgasm*, research shows that they also may enhance your immune system, promote sleep, help prevent heart attacks, reduce stress, provide pain relief, increase pain thresholds, relieve menstrual cramps and migraines, help bring a baby to term in pregnancy, prevent endometriosis, and help decrease your risk of breast cancer. Other research suggests that sex may also help you lose weight, promote reduced blood pressure, lower cholesterol, increase longevity, and improve your sense of well-being.

How Many Ways Can You Have an Orgasm?

Women are multiorgasmic, in more ways than one: the female body is not only able to have repeated orgasms with no refractory period, but is also anatomically blessed with more than a single means of reaching climax. For some women, orgasms come in a variety of styles. How many potential pathways to pleasure do women have? Let us count the ways. . . .

Female orgasms can be clitoral, vaginal, cervical, uterine, or stimulated by the G-spot and culminating in female ejaculation. Clitoral orgasms, probably the most familiar type to many women, are achieved by direct stimulation of the clitoris. Vaginal orgasms typically occur during sex, stimulated by penetration and thrusting of the penis in the vagina. Some women report cervical orgasms—the sensation of orgasm occurring in the cervix, possibly stimulated by deep penetration during sex—although this appears to be far less common than vaginal orgasms. Uterine orgasms appear to be infrequent, too, but some women report sensations of orgasm in the uterus, which may be stimulated by intercourse. Although G-spot ejaculatory orgasms, which we'll explore below, also seem less common, this is partly because they're not yet widely recognized.

Different nerves feed each area of the pelvis, so some women may experience any of these five kinds of orgasms at different times, or perhaps simultaneously—in a "blended orgasm" that involves the nerves and sensations for more than one type of orgasm. Each of the various possible combinations of blended orgasm is arguably a separate type unto itself, so the number of ways women can have orgasms is five at the very least, and perhaps far more.

It's important to realize that there's no "best" type of orgasm for all women. You may want to explore different possible types, but your body is unique, and whichever you experience naturally is right for you. If you have a single type of orgasm, it doesn't mean your sexuality is somehow limited or not fully experienced.

Many women have exclusively clitoral or vaginal orgasms, with such extremes of pleasure-pulsating sensation that they can't imagine wanting anything else. If you're fortunate enough to be orgasmic in the first place, you can't possibly be "missing" anything; an orgasm is a gift and an anatomical miracle, regardless of which kind you experience.

Just as the type of orgasm varies from one woman to the next, so do its distinguishing characteristics. You may climax with fast, frenzied intensity, or have gradual, gentle orgasms that feel as if you're gliding in spectacular slow motion over the edge of a waterfall. Women who experience G-spot ejaculatory orgasms often describe them as deeply intense and cathartic. Again, there's no "right" degree of intensity or universally preferable quality for orgasms—just as every woman certainly doesn't conform to the four phases of the so-called sexual response cycle (*excitement, plateau, orgasm,* and *resolution*) often used to define sexual function—and the best kind of orgasm for you is the kind that your body naturally enjoys.

Female Ejaculation:
The Type of Orgasm That Few Know About

When people hear the phrase *female ejaculation,* they sometimes don't take it seriously—perhaps because they've never experienced it and can't imagine it's possible. It may also be because female ejaculation continues to be poorly understood—or not understood at all—by many in the medical community. It doesn't appear in medical texts or curricula, and you can still find any number of "experts" who insist that it's anatomically impossible, or even that the urethral sponge doesn't exist. This can be frustrating for women who ejaculate during orgasm and have nowhere to turn for information—or confirmation that they're perfectly normal.

As recently as the 1980s, it was difficult to find a single self-help book on sex that even mentioned female ejaculation. Today, although more researchers acknowledge its existence (see accompanying sidebar), books broaching the subject remain few and far between. The shortage of information is no doubt compounded by the fact that not all women ejaculate—or are aware that they do—during orgasm.

Because female ejaculation hasn't yet been adequately elucidated, it deserves extra attention here. Let's look more closely at what happens when a woman ejaculates during orgasm, what leads up to it, and which organs are involved.

Earlier in this chapter we described how to locate your G-spot, and pointed out that it's situated directly over your urethral sponge (your G-sponge). In a sense, your G-spot isn't a separate entity, but simply the place on your vaginal wall where you can most easily reach your G-sponge and stimulate it. Many people don't realize that the G-spot earned its reputation for triggering orgasmic ecstasy only because pressing on it during arousal means directly stimulating the sponge.

As you become aroused, your G-sponge, which contains erectile tissue and glands, becomes engorged, not only with blood but with the fluid it produces. This is why you can most easily find your G-spot during arousal, by reaching your finger inside your vagina to feel your swollen sponge; you can further stimulate its fluid buildup by pressing directly on the spongy surface via your G-spot. Ejaculation happens when intense contractions of the PC muscle during orgasm "squeeze" the built-up fluid in the sponge into the urethra (which the sponge surrounds and presses closely against) and out of the body through the urethral opening.

The fluid that a woman ejaculates, which has been called *amrita,* or "female nectar," has a clear, watery quality and a pleasant, musky smell. It's not easily confused with the vagina's naturally secreted lubrication, and noticeably different from urine. But because it emerges from the urethral opening and many women, as well as many doctors, are unaware that it's produced by paraurethral glands in the G-sponge, it's often mistakenly believed to be urine.

As mentioned previously in this chapter, the G-sponge is sometimes called the female prostate because it's the female counterpart of the male prostate gland, and a woman's ejaculatory fluid resembles male prostatic fluid, although more diluted. It's worth noting that a man's ejaculatory fluid correspondingly contains prostatic fluid, which is produced in his prostate.

Depending on the degree of G-sponge stimulation and the intensity of orgasmic muscle contractions, some women release copious amounts of their female nectar. It can spill out in sudden warm gushes that bathe a woman's vulva, or it can actually squirt like a fountain into the air, projected several inches or more out of her body. Some women release smaller amounts that trickle out less conspicuously.

All women have the potential for ejaculation, but it may require an unusual amount of sexual energy, a high state of arousal, and consistent G-spot stimulation for 20 minutes or longer. When sexual pleasure builds to a sufficient crescendo at orgasm, a woman may arch her back and hold her breath at the point of ejaculation, her pelvic muscles tightening forcefully and propelling her nectar from her body. Some women find that the more G-sponge stimulation they receive, the more ejaculatory they become, and experience multiple ejaculations in sequence without needing a recovery period. It's also possible for a woman to ejaculate before, after, or without any other type of orgasm.

Some women ejaculate naturally, with no extra G-sponge stimulation. Many may do so without realizing it because they're distracted by pleasure, or not adequately in touch with their bodies to recognize what's happening. Many others may be aware of what's going on but concerned that something is "wrong" with them because of the dearth of information on female ejaculation.

The bottom line: If clear fluid is released from your urethral opening when you're aroused—whether it dribbles from your vulva or bursts out like a geyser—you have no cause for fear or alarm. To the contrary, this can be a completely healthy part of your sexual response, and a source of immense pleasure.

> ## Is Female Ejaculation "The New G-Spot"?
>
> In some ways, female ejaculation is to today's generation what the G-spot was to a previous one: an important aspect of female sexuality that many are completely unaware of, few understand, and some consider largely a myth. However, with increasing numbers of women openly describing their experiences of ejaculating, it appears that female ejaculation, once almost a taboo topic among many medical professionals and gynecologists, is finally beginning to emerge from the closet. It seems that it will be just a matter of time, research, and education before it's no longer widely dismissed as impossible. Female ejaculation is real, and here to stay!

Chi and Your Pelvis: The Great Sex Vortex

The ancient wisdom of Chinese medicine has a lot to say about your pelvis and sexual health. As you've discovered, your pelvis plays a pivotal role as the conduit for all the chi that courses through your body in channels known as meridians. You can nourish your sexuality, resolve many pelvic-health issues, and boost your general health by keeping your chi abundant and flowing smoothly through your pelvis. By following all the steps outlined in Chapters 1 and 2 for creating a sturdy foundation of health, you can keep your chi strong.

If your chi isn't flowing efficiently, you can develop what's known as "stuck chi" in your pelvis. This can be caused by poor general health, or emotional issues such as unresolved anger or grief from abuse, miscarriages, or abortions. If you have stuck chi in your pelvis, your meridians can't bring vital energy to your pelvic organs, and you're prone to forming masses such as fibroids and ovarian cysts. Stuck chi in your pelvis can also result in abnormal functioning of your pelvic organs, pain, or reduction in the quality of your sex life.

Your pelvis is an energetic vortex because it concentrates not only your chi, but also a special form of chi that originates in your kidneys. For the purposes of this book, we call this type of chi your *sexual chi* because of its unique, primal connection to your sexuality. According to Chinese medicine, your sexual chi fills your meridians and has powerful therapeutic effects on your

61

entire body, mind, and spirit. For example, it increases your circulation, nurtures your emotions, and reinforces your overall chi. Because of your sexual chi, loving sex that deeply bonds you with your partner has profound healing effects on many levels.

Your sexual chi can be especially healing to the organs and tissues of your pelvis, by flushing your female organs with energy, blood, oxygen, and nutrition. You need abundant sexual chi to maintain a robust sexual appetite; if it's low, intimacy won't hold much attraction for you. Chinese medicine teaches that common problems with sex organs, such as chronic vaginal infections, ovarian cysts, or painful menstrual cycles, can be resolved by restoring sexual chi.

You can enhance your capacity for great sex—or replenish your sexual energy if it's depleted—by tapping into the power of your sexual chi. Because your sexual chi is derived from your entire body, mind, and spirit, you can build it with lifestyle shifts that improve your health and happiness. A balanced lifestyle gives you ample sexual chi, but a life of excess quickly depletes it. As with your overall chi, following the recommendations earlier in this book for creating a strong foundation of health will cultivate your sexual chi.

You can also stimulate your sexual chi with acupressure. Your body stores a vast reservoir of it in your pelvis, at an acupressure point called *Ren 6,* also known as the *Sea of Chi.* Another point for enhancing sexual chi, called *Kidney 1* (also known as *Gushing Spring* because it's traditionally considered an upward-flowing fountain of energy), is found on your foot. To locate both points on your body, see Appendix A. By pressing firmly on these points for a few minutes each day, you can strengthen your sexual chi.

Getting into Your Flow with Acupressure

According to Chinese medicine, you can directly affect the channels of chi that flow through your body by pressing on key points along the courses they follow. When you stimulate your chi with acupressure, it can have systemic effects on your body, mind, spirit, and sexual energy. Acupressure can be thought of as a variation on acupuncture that you can easily apply yourself. To do so, you use your finger to press gently but firmly on a designated point for one to three minutes. This simple technique of applying steady pressure to the point enhances the flow of your chi through it.

"Sex-Flex" Exercises for Boosting Pleasure and Empowering Your Pelvis

You can create greater pelvic health and increase your sexual satisfaction by strengthening, firming, stretching, and releasing your pelvic muscles. Exercises for enhancing sex and boosting pelvic-muscle strength have been recommended in Chinese medicine for centuries. One well-known Chinese manual, *The Art of the Bedchamber,* instructed women to exercise their pelvic muscles and improve vaginal sensation with "pelvic squeezing" during sex.

According to traditional Chinese medicine, strengthening your pelvic muscles brings chi to your pelvis and improves its flow throughout your body. In addition, if your pelvic muscles are weak and lack tone, your vagina "leaks" your sexual chi, resulting in a reduced sex drive and overall fatigue. When your pelvic muscles are strong, they preserve the healing force of your sexual chi, and use it to maximize the health of your female organs.

The best-known modern exercises for enhancing pleasure and pelvic strength are Kegels. Introduced in the 1940s by physician Arnold Kegel to treat urinary incontinence (the involuntary release of urine), the exercises had the unexpected benefit of also improving women's sex lives; some who did them regularly reported having orgasms for the first time.

Kegels increase blood flow to your pelvis and keep you connected with your core by familiarizing you with your inner pelvic muscles, particularly your PC muscle. By learning how to contract and relax your PC muscle, you can increase the intensity of your orgasms and literally flex your way to better sex—and also enhance your partner's pleasure by increasing his sensation as your vagina tightens around his penis.

In addition to preventing and treating urinary incontinence, which we'll explore later in this chapter, doing Kegels on a regular basis can prevent, alleviate, or reverse pelvic organ prolapse, which occurs if your pelvis doesn't correctly support an organ. Kegels help with this condition by lifting, toning, and building up your inner pelvic muscles, which (as described in previous pages) include the PC muscle that forms the "hammock" holding up your pelvic organs. This is why Kegels are recommended for women about to give birth, or recovering from a vaginal birth. A

63

woman's pelvic muscles expand dramatically during childbirth, and afterward can remain stretched and weakened, making her prone to organ prolapse.

You can do Kegels slowly, which develops your slow-twitch muscle fibers, builds your strength and stamina, and promotes your overall pelvic-muscle tone. You can also do them rapidly, which fortifies your fast-twitch fibers. The best results are usually achieved by combining the slow and fast techniques, with more emphasis on the slow.

To do a Kegel, you tighten the muscles you would use if you were trying to stop your flow of urine. (If necessary, try this while urinating; you won't want to do it often, but experimenting a few times will acquaint you with the muscles you need to use, and what it feels like to contract them.) You're ready to begin doing Kegels when you've learned to contract and relax these muscles.

For starters, here's a simple Kegel routine you can try: do fast Kegels for two seconds, rest for two seconds, and repeat eight to ten times; then do a slow Kegel that lasts for ten seconds, relax for ten seconds, and repeat eight to ten times. You can do this routine several times a day at your convenience. One of the beauties of Kegels is that they can be done in practically any position—sitting, standing, or lying down—so you can privately practice your "sex flex" almost anytime and anywhere. You can do your Kegels while waiting in line at the store, sitting on a plane, or stuck in traffic. Stoplights were made for them!

Keep practicing this basic routine, and you'll become a proficient Kegeler before you know it. Later in this book, we'll explore some exciting advanced techniques that incorporate the use of special cones and weighted devices known as Ben Wa balls, which were first developed in ancient China.

Most women have little trouble mastering Kegels, but some find it difficult to identify and flex their PC muscle. If you're in this category, the guidance of a physical therapist trained in biofeedback to promote PC-muscle strength can be enormously helpful. A biofeedback probe inserted into your vagina allows you to gauge the duration and strength of your PC contractions. (You can also purchase at-home biofeedback devices, such as the Pelvic Muscle Therapy Program, for under $50.) If you experience spasms or difficulty releasing your inner pelvic muscles, devices known as *vaginal dilators,* available online or through your physical therapist, can help.

Enhancing Your Sexuality by Solving Common Pelvic Problems

You may need to enhance your experience of sex because of a particular health challenge you face with your pelvis or sexual organs. If you've had trouble enjoying sexual pleasure or achieving an orgasm, either by yourself or with a partner, you're not alone; thousands of women have similar experiences. The good news is that you can overcome many common pelvic- and sexual-health issues, and it can be extremely empowering to discover that you can increase your own capacity for sexual gratification via natural means.

Problems that interfere with sexual enjoyment can have both psychological and physical causes. The psychological causes include untreated anxiety and depression, chronic long-term stress, a history of sexual abuse or trauma, issues pertaining to body image, and self-esteem issues. Women who fear intimacy, or don't trust their partner enough to release control and allow themselves to have an orgasm, are more prone to sexual difficulties and less likely to experience pleasure in a relationship.

If you have sexual challenges with psychological causes, whatever the issue may be, a therapist can help you uncover patterns in your behavior that may be blocking you from your natural ability to experience sexual satisfaction. With time, you can work through inhibitions you may have about sex.

The physical causes of an unsatisfactory sex life can include painful menstrual cramps; chronic pelvic infections known as *vaginitis;* vaginal atrophy and dryness (the decrease in size, reduced elasticity, thinning, or increased fragility of tissue that often happens in midlife); urinary incontinence; urinary tract infections; interstitial cystitis; ovarian disorders such as benign cysts or polycystic ovarian syndrome; cervical dysplasia; chronic pelvic pain; and hormone imbalances (which we'll explore in detail in the next chapter). Some prescription medications, such as

65

antidepressants, blood-pressure medications, and antihistamines, can also decrease your libido and inhibit orgasm.

If you have a condition that prevents you from fully enjoying sex, remember that you are your own expert on your sexuality—the only person with direct experience of your body, mind, and spirit, and intimate knowledge of your entire personal history—and that you can resolve many common problems of the pelvis and sexual organs without drugs or medical intervention. In the pages ahead, you'll discover numerous ways you can enhance your capacity for pleasure with safe, natural self-help solutions to the sexual-health challenges you're most likely to face.

Enabling Pleasure:
Getting Past Painful Menstrual Cramps

You may be surprised to discover that you don't necessarily have to live through painful menstrual cramping every month. One of the great myths about women's health in conventional medicine is that menstrual cramps are inevitable—and that it's perfectly acceptable to take anti-inflammatory drugs or over-the-counter medications like Midol every month to treat the symptoms. By challenging this view and using natural means to alleviate menstrual cramps, you stand a good chance of having pain-free periods—and a time of month you may have once written off as invariably uncomfortable can instead become an opportunity for more pleasurable pursuits.

If you have painful menstruation, or *dysmenorrhea,* you know it usually happens during the first two to three days of your period. The cramping you experience may be partly due to changes in your hormones and your body's production of "unfriendly" prostaglandins (hormone-like substances). Some women have painful menstrual cramping because of unusual conditions such as pelvic inflammatory disease, uterine fibroids, ovarian cysts, or other health issues. If you're not in this category and your cramping is "normal," the following natural methods are likely to significantly reduce or eliminate your discomfort:

— **Western herbs.** Ginger and cramp bark (also known by its botanical name, *Viburnum opulus*) are among the best Western herbs for decreasing menstrual pain. Ginger is most effective as a tea; to relieve cramping, drink three or four cups a day, beginning when your period starts and continuing as needed. Cramp-bark capsules are available in many health-food stores; the recommended dose is 300 mg three times daily.

— **Chinese herbal formulas.** According to Chinese medicine, menstrual cramps are typically caused by "chi and blood stagnation," which is associated with feelings of stress and frustration. One of the best-known formulas for the condition, Xiao Yao Wan (also known as *Free and Easy Wanderer*), is available at some health-food stores and online; for dosage, follow the recommendations on the product label.

— **Omega-3 fatty acids.** Omega-3 fatty acids can relieve menstrual cramps by helping your body make more "friendly" prostaglandins that reduce pain and inflammation. They are found in fish oil, flax oil, and walnuts.

— **Magnesium citrate.** For many women, this is a reliable treatment for menstrual cramps. The most effective dose is 600 mg taken a few days before the onset of your period, and continued through the first three days of your period. (Note: Excessive magnesium intake can cause diarrhea.)

— **Other supplements.** To help keep the cramping away, make sure you're also getting 400 IU of vitamin E and 1,000 mg of calcium every day.

67

— **Exercise.** There's conflicting research on whether exercise helps reduce menstrual pain, but anecdotal evidence strongly suggests that it can. For many women, a workout a day keeps the cramping away! From the Chinese medical perspective, exercise may resolve menstrual cramps by increasing the circulation of chi in your pelvis and preventing stagnation. You may want to try different kinds of exercise before and during your period to see what works best for you.

— **Acupressure.** You can also use acupressure to relieve menstrual cramps. At the onset of cramping, you or your partner can press gently on the point known as *Spleen 6* and hold for one to three minutes, at least once per hour as needed. To locate this point on your body, see Appendix A.

— **Regular sex.** For some women, having sex regularly during the rest of the month (when they're not menstruating) can help alleviate menstrual cramps.

Natural Sex-Enhancing Treatments for Vaginitis

If you have vaginitis, or an inflammation or infection of your vagina, it can seriously interfere with your sex life. Chronic vaginal infections, which are among the most common sexual-health challenges women experience, are often accompanied by pain and itching in both the vagina and vulva. In some cases, there may be only irritation at the vaginal opening; in others, there may also be a vaginal discharge. Overcoming this condition can be extremely liberating, and dramatically enhance your sexuality.

Your vagina has its own dynamic ecology that's influenced by your lifestyle, diet, immune system, hormones, and other factors. Various microorganisms inhabit your vagina, including both "friendly" and "unfriendly" bacteria and yeast. When you're healthy, your vagina is naturally self-cleansing and self-regulating; your friendly bacteria hold the unfriendly bacteria and yeast at bay and help keep your vaginal pH (its degree of acidity or alkalinity) at a level that assists in preventing infections.

If you have vaginitis, it's most likely due to an overgrowth of unfriendly bacteria or yeast. This can happen if you disrupt your vaginal balance by consuming too much sugar or taking too many antibiotics. Unnecessary douching to diminish so-called feminine odors can also make your vagina more vulnerable to infections. In addition, vaginitis can be caused by too much of a good thing: frequent sex can change the pH of your vaginal environment and allow unfriendly bacteria to thrive, because the pH of semen is more alkaline than that of your vagina.

To identify the cause of vaginitis, you need to see a physician for an accurate diagnosis. Although usually the result of an overgrowth of unfriendly bacteria or yeast, it can also be due to a sexually transmitted infection such as trichomoniasis, which is caused by a microscopic parasite. If you have trichomoniasis, you'll need to take an antibiotic, and your partner will as well.

Many conventional physicians, unaware that you can treat and prevent vaginitis caused by unfriendly bacteria or yeast with natural methods, are far too quick to prescribe drugs that can be counterproductive and further disrupt your vaginal balance. For example, women are frequently prescribed antibiotics for bacterial infections in the vagina, but this often destroys not only the unfriendly bacteria that caused the infection but also the friendly bacteria that could have prevented it from recurring. Antibiotics may seem like a short-term fix, but they often contribute to infections returning.

To treat vaginitis due to unfriendly bacteria or yeast, you want to use natural treatments whenever possible and lifestyle changes that affect your entire body, not just your vagina. If you have chronic vaginitis due to yeast, for instance, you should eat a diet low in sugar, alcohol, and refined carbohydrates. You should also make lifestyle changes such as removing a wet bathing suit soon after swimming (leaving it on could make you more prone to vaginal yeast infection), and avoiding clothing that fits tightly around your lower pelvis; one study showed that you can be three times more likely to experience vaginitis if you wear panty hose.

Let's look at the most effective natural methods you can use to treat vaginitis caused by overgrowth of unfriendly bacteria or yeast:

— **Vaginal douche powder.** One of the best natural medicines I've prescribed for vaginal bacterial and yeast imbalances is a vaginal douche powder called Tanafem (to obtain it, see Appendix C) consisting of zinc tannates and glycine. It eradicates bacteria and yeast by dehydrating them, and you can get rid of most infections by using it twice daily for a week. Soothing and nonirritating, it can even be applied to reddened, highly inflamed tissues. Mix one scoop in a pint-size douche bag filled with warm water, and douche twice daily for five to ten days, depending on the severity of the infection.

Using vaginal douche powder in conjunction with a sitz bath can help alleviate any external irritation you may have. (A *sitz bath* is a German term for sitting in a bowl of water to heal and nurture the tissues of the pelvis, or to increase circulation through the pelvis. Many irritations of the vulva can be treated with sitz baths.) Mix one scoop of the powder with warm water in a pan large enough for you to be seated comfortably; place the pan on the floor, and soak your vulva in this bath for 10 to 20 minutes twice a day for five to ten days, depending on the degree of inflammation. (Note: The rust-colored powder may permanently stain the pan, towels, and bath mats.)

— **Tea-tree oil.** An effective treatment for overgrowth of unfriendly bacteria or yeast, tea-tree oil can be used either as a douche or in the form of vaginal suppositories. (If your vagina is inflamed to the point of being "raw" and red, tea-tree oil shouldn't be used, as it could be irritating.) For douching, mix ten drops of oil in a pint of warm water and douche; do this twice daily for seven to ten days. For suppositories, place one tea-tree oil suppository in your vagina twice a day for seven to ten days. You may want to wear a menstrual pad, as the oil from the suppositories can leak out.

You can purchase tea-tree-oil vaginal suppositories online or at your local natural-health pharmacy. They're typically made with cocoa butter or vitamin E, which can be soothing to your vaginal mucosa—your vagina's protective outer layer of moist tissue. Keep them on hand, and use one whenever you feel the beginning of a vaginal infection; this can nip it in the bud, preventing full-blown vaginitis.

— **Goldenseal root.** Also known as *hydrastis,* goldenseal can be used as a douche, as a sitz bath, or as vaginal suppositories to treat vaginal infections. It's antibacterial, antifungal (which means it kills yeast), and gentle on your tissues. You can find goldenseal root at most herbal dispensaries, often as a powder, capsule, or pill. If you purchase capsules, you can open them and use the contents to make the mixture for your douche or sitz bath.

For a douche or sitz bath, bring four cups of water to a boil, add a tablespoon of goldenseal root, simmer for 15 minutes, strain, and let cool until it's at a warm temperature, comfortable to douche with or sit in. For douching, use this mixture to douche twice daily for a week. For sitz baths, warm the mixture, pour it into a large pan, and sit in the pan for 10 minutes twice daily for two days.

To use goldenseal vaginal suppositories, place one in your vagina twice daily for a week. You may need to obtain goldenseal suppositories through your naturopathic physician; the ones I recommend, which are in a base of cocoa butter, are well tolerated by most women.

— **Chinese herbal wash.** You can treat vaginitis caused by bacteria or yeast, and nurture this sensitive yin area of your body with an antipathogenic herbal remedy from a Chinese-herb store. The product Yin-care combines a number of organic Chinese herbs, and makes an effective douche; for information on obtaining it, see Appendix C. Yin-care is recommended for chronic vaginal imbalances, known as "damp heat" conditions in the terminology of traditional Chinese medicine.

For douching, dilute the herbal wash in warm water, following the directions on the product label, and douche twice daily for five days. If you have a chronic or severe infection, mix the herbal wash with an equal amount of water, soak a tampon in the solution, place the tampon in your vagina, and leave it there for three hours; do this twice daily for six days.

— **Friendly bacteria vaginal suppositories.** If you suffer from bacterial vaginitis, you need to restore your vagina's bacterial balance with friendly bacteria. Your vagina is healthiest when your friendly bacteria keep the unfriendly elements in check and help maintain your vaginal pH at the right level.

You can purchase over-the-counter suppositories containing friendly vaginal bacteria, known as *Lactobacillus acidophilus,* but it's important not to overuse them; you don't want an overgrowth of friendly bacteria. For most chronic or acute vaginal infections, use one suppository a week for seven weeks. (See Appendix C for information on purchasing friendly bacteria vaginal suppositories.)

71

To help determine whether vaginitis is caused by bacteria, examine any discharge you may have. If it's yellow-green with a slightly fishy odor, you most likely have a bacterial infection; if it's white and curd-like, you probably have a vaginal yeast infection. For a definitive diagnosis, however, you'll need to see a doctor.

— Cleansing. You can have chronic vaginitis from bacteria or yeast if your immune system isn't in peak form and your overall health is compromised. Many women with chronic vaginitis also have excessive yeast or unfriendly bacteria in their intestines, the result of an overwhelmed immune system that can't rally to restore balance between friendly and unfriendly bacteria and yeast. With your Great Sex Detox, the cleanse outlined in Chapter 2, you can recharge the health of your entire body and effectively eradicate vaginitis.

Facilitating Sex: Solutions for Vaginal Dryness and VAD

Vaginal dryness is one of the most disconcerting sexual-health challenges you may face. Most women experience it to one degree or another at some time in their lives. If you have vaginal dryness, there's no mistaking the symptoms, especially if you experience it during sex; insufficient lubrication can be debilitating to your sex life. One woman graphically described the condition to me as "a sensation that my vaginal walls are lined with sandpaper." Another summed it up as "feeling like I have dust bunnies in my vagina." Solving vaginal dryness can be one of the most sex-enhancing steps you ever take.

If you experience vaginal dryness at any time in your life, you can benefit immeasurably by using natural lubricants as needed for sex. We'll cover many of your options for sexual lubricants in detail later in this book.

When vaginal dryness is accompanied by the thinning of the tissue of the vulva and vagina known as *atrophy,* which often happens during midlife, the condition is referred to as *vulvovaginal atrophy* or *vaginal atrophy and dryness* (which we call *VAD*). The name may sound clinical, but it describes an experience that for many women is all too real. VAD is a silent epidemic that affects millions of women, including up to 60 percent of those in their postmenopausal years.

Your vaginal and vulvar tissues naturally secrete sex-enhancing lubrication, and the secret to your secretions often lies in your estrogen level. VAD is caused by the natural reduction of estrogen throughout your body as you approach midlife; the tissues of your vulva and vagina are uniquely sensitive to this decrease because they're estrogen-dependent. The drop in estrogen can decrease blood flow to these tissues, and lower their collagen content, and since collagen makes up your connective tissue, this means more tissue breakdown and atrophy. In addition to atrophy, the most noticeable effect of VAD is the reduction of your natural lubrication, and vulvar or vaginal pain that can last for months, or years.

If you have VAD, you may also experience vaginal irritation, itching, tenderness, urinary incontinence, and pain or bleeding during sex. Your symptoms can range from uncomfortable to excruciating, and sex may be out of the question. You may visit a number of gynecologists who prescribe topical steroid creams and vaginal anti-yeast creams—all to no avail. You may conclude that nothing can be done, and resolve to live with your symptoms.

Although both vaginal dryness and VAD are among the most common challenges women experience, VAD is one of the least recognized. There has been a tendency to downplay or ignore it in conventional medicine, which provides no clear explanation for why some women have the condition and some don't. Since VAD often begins when a woman is in her 40s and continues into postmenopause, conventional doctors sometimes consider it just another unpleasant change that comes with the territory of midlife, a "minor" affliction requiring no special medical attention.

If untreated, VAD can lead to numerous other conditions, including vaginitis. Low estrogen in your vaginal tissues can make you more vulnerable to pH shifts and vaginal infections from unwanted bacteria and yeast. This happens because your vagina and urethra are lined with *mucosa*—the protective, moist outer barrier that lubricates your tissues and helps prevent vaginal infections from bacteria and yeast, as well as urinary tract infections. When the estrogen level in these tissues drops and your urethral and vaginal tissues become thinner and more fragile with atrophy, your protective mucosal barrier can break down, increasing the potential for bacteria or yeast invasion.

If you suffer from vaginal dryness or VAD, the good news is that there are many ways you can alleviate your symptoms, and you may be able to make them disappear completely. Treating VAD often means mitigating its effects by nourishing and supporting your vulvar and vaginal tissues.

From the perspective of traditional Chinese medicine, the symptoms of vaginal dryness and VAD are by no means an inevitable part of your life; they're seen as the result of an imbalance in your chi, and inadequate circulation of chi through your pelvis. The underlying causes can be treated with herbs, some blended in ancient formulas that give them synergistic effects—which means they're more effective in combination than alone. Two of these formulas, included below, can be used to balance your chi, enhance your overall health, and nurture your vulvar and vaginal tissues.

For many women—especially those with severe dryness and great discomfort—using any one treatment alone may not provide the entire solution to VAD. Some find that combining Western methods, such as topical estrogen cream and vitamin E, works best, while others find a blend of Western and Chinese methods most effective. And for many, combining treatments with the lifestyle changes we've covered earlier in this book, along with Kegels or other exercises for increasing blood flow to their vaginal tissues, helps treat the underlying deficiency and create change on a deeper level. If you suffer from vaginal dryness or VAD, a multifaceted approach that incorporates lifestyle changes will not only enhance your sexuality by nurturing the tissues of your vulva and vagina, but also build your libido by boosting your overall health.

Let's look at the most effective natural methods you can use to reduce or eliminate the effects of vaginal dryness and VAD, including three treatments from Chinese medicine. (Note: If you have vaginal dryness but you don't have VAD, the first two methods—estrogen creams and DHEA suppositories—aren't recommended, but the others are.)

— **Natural estrogen creams.** By using a low-dose natural estrogen cream on your vulva and in your vagina, you can rehydrate your tissues, enhance their integrity, and support your urethra.

It's recommended that you use the lowest possible dose of the cream needed. If you have a history of breast cancer or other cancer linked to estrogen, you shouldn't use an estrogen cream, since even a low dose can stimulate estrogen-related cancer growth.

The best natural estrogen cream to use contains *estriol,* a type of estrogen that's much weaker than estradiol and other estrogens commonly used in hormone replacement therapy. As the primary estrogen produced by the body during pregnancy, estriol is "friendlier" than estradiol, and can't convert in your body into stronger forms of estrogen.

Not only can estriol make an enormous difference in VAD by enhancing the integrity of your protective mucosa and allowing for more lubrication during sex, but it can also help prevent urinary tract infections, which can be common during the years leading up to menopause. In addition, by strengthening the tissues of your urethra, estriol can help prevent urinary incontinence—a common condition in menopausal women who experience VAD.

To use estriol vaginal cream, apply a dose of 2 mg nightly before bed for ten nights by placing a small amount on your fingertip; gently spread the cream on your vulva and in your vagina. After ten nights, taper to 1 mg nightly three times a week. (You can also apply it with a vaginal applicator, if the cream you use comes with one.) After following this protocol for as little as a few weeks, many women report that they no longer experience vulvar or vaginal discomfort, and can have pain-free sex once again.

As an alternative, you can use estriol in the form of vaginal suppositories, which are used much like the cream and in similar doses, except that you insert the suppositories into your vagina. Neither the cream nor the suppositories are available over-the-counter; they're by prescription only, and should be used under the direction of a licensed naturopathic physician or other qualified holistic doctor.

Since some of the estriol you apply will be absorbed into your system, it's highly recommended that you use a small amount of natural progesterone simultaneously. This helps to balance the effect of the estriol and prevent the unwanted buildup of the *endometrium,* or inner lining of your uterus. (If you've had a hysterectomy, this isn't applicable.) In the next chapter, we'll explore in detail what you need to know about taking progesterone.

— DHEA suppositories. If you can't use estrogen, you can use the hormone DHEA in the form of vaginal suppositories. This can effectively increase your vaginal moisture and resolve symptoms of VAD, especially if you have vaginal atrophy, without increasing your risk of tissue overgrowth in the inner lining of your uterus that could lead to endometrial cancer.

A 2009 study published in the journal *Menopause* found that menopausal women with vaginal atrophy who used DHEA vaginal suppositories showed significant improvements in their vaginal symptoms, which included pain during sex, dryness, irritation, and itching. And after three months of using the suppositories, they had no increase in endometrial growth.

To use DHEA vaginal suppositories, insert a 5 mg suppository into your vagina every night before you go to bed. DHEA vaginal suppositories are available by prescription only. (Note: Women with a history of estrogen-related cancer shouldn't use DHEA.)

— Black-cohosh and wild-yam suppositories. A gentler way to enhance your vulvar and vaginal integrity is with vaginal suppositories containing both black cohosh and wild yam in a natural cocoa-butter base. These can be the answer for vaginal dryness, and a wonderful solution to VAD if you'd rather not use estriol, or any kind of hormone. (They can also be an effective add-on if you use estriol or DHEA, but they don't completely solve VAD.) Typically, these suppositories also contain some vitamin E.

Although the herb black cohosh doesn't contain any estrogen, it has active constituents that may have estrogen-like effects on your tissues and can help increase vulvar and vaginal lubrication. Black cohosh has been used by naturopathic doctors for decades to help women through the changes they experience in the years leading up to and beyond midlife. It's often taken as a pill to help with hot flashes and other symptoms associated with low estrogen.

Wild yam contains active compounds that have progesterone-like effects—and also contains ingredients that have estrogen-like effects. Like black cohosh, it contains no hormones but can give you many of the same benefits.

To use the suppositories, insert one into your vagina every night at bedtime; after two weeks, taper use to two or three times a week to enhance lubrication. For many women, the suppositories are helpful within one or two weeks of use. (See Appendix C for supplier information.) If you have a history of breast cancer, you may be able to use black-cohosh and wild-yam suppositories, but you should check with your doctor first.

— **Vitamin E.** The unique properties of vitamin E make it especially effective for relieving vaginal dryness and VAD, stimulating your normal mucosa, and decreasing the potential for infection. As with black-cohosh and wild-yam suppositories, vitamin E can also be helpful if you use estriol or DHEA, and if they don't fully resolve symptoms of VAD.

For an easy home remedy, open a soft 400 IU vitamin E gel capsule with a pin, squeeze the oil onto your fingertip, and apply it directly to your vulva and vaginal tissues. (Vitamin E is also available in liquid form. It's always best to purchase vitamin E in the form of mixed tocopherols.)

Vitamin E can also reduce vaginal dryness when used as a suppository. The vitamin E vaginal suppository in Appendix C is available in a natural cocoa-butter base that melts at body temperature after you apply it, allowing the vitamin E to cover the tissues of your vulva and vagina. To use, insert one suppository into your vagina with your finger.

Whether you use vitamin E gel capsules or vitamin E vaginal suppositories, you should apply them every night at bedtime for at least two weeks, then taper use to three times a week to keep your vulvar and vaginal tissues hydrated. Many women with vaginal dryness or VAD begin to experience an improvement in their symptoms after using one of these treatments for only a week or two.

For the most effective relief of vaginal dryness experienced during sex, use one of these methods long-term and on a regular basis. Either can also be used before or during sex as a lubricant, although you'll probably find that the suppositories result in much smoother, more effective lubrication than the gel capsules. In either case, a panty liner is recommended; vitamin E oil may be staining.

— **Ba Zhen Wan.** Also referred to as "Women's Precious Pills" or "Women's Eight Treasure Tea Pills," Ba Zhen Wan strengthens a type of chi known as *Xue*. According to Chinese medicine, if you have an imbalance of Xue, your symptoms may include vulvar and vaginal tissues that are pale, undernourished, and devitalized, as well as a faded complexion, heart palpitations, shortness of breath, weak feelings in your limbs, dizziness, a pale tongue, and a faint pulse. (From the perspective of Western medicine, this state may be associated with anemia, painful menstrual cramps, low blood sugar, ulcers or abscesses that don't heal, and postpartum exhaustion.)

Ba Zhen Wan contains five herbs that work synergistically to balance your chi: *poria, licorice, ligusticum, white-peony root,* and *Angelica sinensis.* The recommended dose is two pills two to three times daily, or if in pellet form, eight pellets two to three times daily. (Many companies make Chinese herbal formulas in both pill and pellet form. The pills are larger, approximately five to eight millimeters lengthwise; the small round pellets, or *BBs,* are typically about three millimeters in diameter.) See Appendix C for a resource.

You can also use acupressure to complement the effects of Ba Zhen Wan and help balance your chi: press firmly on the point called *Liver 8* for two minutes once or twice daily. (To locate Liver 8, see Appendix A.)

— **Liu Wei Di Huang Wan.** Also known as "Six Flavor Tea Pills," Liu Wei Di Huang Wan is a Chinese herbal formula that builds another type of chi known as *kidney and liver yin.* It's used for symptoms that include dry, thinning, or burning vulvar and vaginal tissues, as well as for dry skin, night sweats, hot flashes, hot sensations in the palms of the hands and in the feet, blurred vision, dizziness, ringing in the ears, dark circles under the eyes, constipation, a lack of restful sleep, mental unrest, and frequent urination. A woman with these symptoms also tends to have a dry, reddish tongue and a pulse described in Chinese medicine as "thin"—weak and difficult to feel, as opposed to strong and "full." (From the standpoint of Western medicine, this condition may be associated with insomnia, perimenopause and menopause, hyperthyroidism, interstitial cystitis, and other health issues.)

Some research has found that Liu Wei Di Huang Wan can increase the release of adrenal hormones that reduce inflammation; other research has shown it can support and balance immune-system functions. The formula combines six synergistic herbs: *rehmannia, fructus corni, moutan, dioscoreae, poria,* and *alismatis.* The recommended dose is two pills two to three times daily, or (in pellet form) eight pellets two to three times daily.

To use acupressure to support Liu Wei Di Huang Wan and help balance your chi, press firmly on the point called *Spleen 6* (see Appendix A) for two minutes once or twice daily.

— **Chinese ginseng.** You can use Chinese ginseng, also known as *Panax ginseng* or *Korean ginseng,* as a single herb to treat or prevent vaginal dryness or atrophy of your vulvar and vaginal tissues. (Later in this book, you'll explore Chinese ginseng's aphrodisiac effects.) Well known in Chinese medicine for its ability to "build yang," it can be especially effective if you not only have vaginal dryness or VAD but also what's known as "yang deficiency." Symptoms of yang deficiency include cold hands and feet, low energy and vitality, low libido, achy joints, sensations of cold in the lower back and knees, and a lack of control of the flow of urine. (From a Western medical perspective, this condition may be associated with arthritis, fatigue, hypothyroidism, adrenal fatigue, obesity, urinary incontinence, depression, and other ailments.)

Chinese ginseng can improve the circulation of chi through your pelvic region, warm and nurture your pelvic tissues, and help maintain the health and vitality of this delicate area of your body. The recommended dose is 200 mg taken two to three times daily. Since Chinese ginseng is a stimulating herb, it may cause insomnia in some women if taken too late in the day.

To use acupressure to support Chinese ginseng and help balance your chi, press firmly on the point called *San Jiao 4* (see Appendix A) for two minutes once or twice daily.

Providing for Pleasure by Preventing and Treating Urinary Incontinence

Urinary incontinence, or the involuntary release of urine from the bladder, is largely a female affliction; women are five times more likely than men to experience it. Each year, the condition affects many millions of women worldwide. There's more than one type of urinary incontinence, but the most common type that you may experience, known as *stress incontinence,* can be prevented or treated naturally. (We'll address this type here; other types, beyond the scope of this book, require medical attention.) Preventing or treating this condition can vastly improve your ability to enjoy your sexuality.

If you're a woman with the typical case of urinary incontinence, you're unable to prevent urine from leaking out of your urethra when pressure is exerted on your abdomen. This can happen often, since the degree of pressure it takes to cause leakage may happen when you sneeze, cough, lift heavy objects, exercise, squat, jump, or laugh. Leakage may also occur during sex, which can put a damper, literally, on your sex life. The condition can be mild, causing an occasional minor embarrassment, or severe, with consequences drastically affecting the quality of your life.

Urinary incontinence can have many causes, but the most common is childbirth. As you discovered earlier in this chapter, after childbirth a woman's pelvic muscles can remain stretched and weakened, making her more vulnerable to organ prolapse. This can also increase her susceptibility to urinary incontinence.

Another potential cause is the natural hormonal changes you experience leading up to menopause. As the estrogen and testosterone levels in your body decline, some of the tissues in your pelvic muscles, including those that support your bladder and urethra, may become weaker, making them less able to prevent leakage. At the same time, your dropping estrogen level affects estrogen receptors in your nerve tissue in ways that can elevate sensitivity and lead to increased urge to urinate.

Kegels can be effective not only for preventing urinary incontinence but also for treating it; they strengthen and firm the muscles that support your lower pelvis, urethra, and bladder. Earlier in this chapter we described how to do Kegels, and you may already be well on your way to becoming a master Kegeler. Keep practicing the recommended routine, whether or not you have urinary incontinence: you may prevent it from ever developing— or be surprised by how successfully you can reverse the symptoms. Rapid Kegels, which develop the fast-twitch fibers in your pelvic muscles, can be especially helpful in preventing urinary incontinence triggered by sudden abdominal pressure like coughing or sneezing. If you're one of the many women who suffer from urinary incontinence, give extra attention to your fast-Kegel skills.

Freeing Your Libido from Urinary Tract Infections

There's a good chance you've had a urinary tract infection (UTI) at some point in your life. They're among the most common female health concerns, affecting millions of women every year. You may have experienced recurring UTIs; about 20 percent of women who have a UTI have a second one, and some 30 percent of those women have a third.

Women often develop UTIs after having sex, as a result of tissue irritation at the urethral opening or vagina, which is why UTIs are sometimes referred to as "honeymoon cystitis." (In this context, *cystitis* is a term linked with some types of UTIs.) Many women with UTIs are repeatedly prescribed antibiotics by conventional doctors. This may cause their symptoms to disappear for a time, only to return again when they have sex. Antibiotics are sometimes necessary, but when too quickly prescribed, they can contribute to the development of UTIs by killing off the friendly bacteria in your vagina, vulva, and urethra that help prevent UTIs.

Every day, you're exposed to the type of bacteria that causes UTIs. You normally fight them off, but a number of factors can make you more susceptible and allow them to invade your urethra and bladder. In addition to tissue irritation from sex and the inappropriate use of antibiotics, common causes of UTIs include dehydration, general stress on your immune system, and your dietary choices.

UTIs are unpleasant, and can wreak havoc on your sex life because their disagreeable symptoms can cause apprehension about recurrent infections. Symptoms include pain or burning sensations while urinating, pressure in your bladder or urethra, an urgency to urinate, frequent urination, and blood in the urine. The good news is that there's a lot that you can do to assist your body in naturally preventing UTIs, and thereby enormously enhance your ability to enjoy sex. Let's look at the lifestyle measures you can take to help keep yourself UTI-free:

— **Use adequate lubrication during sex.** This can make all the difference in whether or not your vulvar tissues become irritated. Later in this book, we'll explore your options for using sexual lubricants in detail.

— **Urinate after you have sex.** UTIs may gain a foothold in your urethra during sex; with this simple preventive measure, you decrease their chances. Emptying your bladder naturally cleanses unwanted bacteria from your urethra and bladder.

— **Drink plenty of water.** This prevents dehydration, helps keep your tissues moisturized (including your vaginal tissues), and gives you the advantage over undesirable bacteria. Your daily intake of water in ounces should equal about half the weight of your body in pounds, but you may need more in a hot climate, or if you perspire a lot from exercise—or from sex.

— **Choose the right diet.** Avoid sugar and alcohol, both of which can make you more UTI-prone. A diet high in sugar can make you especially vulnerable. Following the Great Sex Diet outlined in Chapter 2 will help you steer clear of UTIs.

— **Avoid using soap on your urethra.** Soap can irritate your delicate vulvar tissue, change its pH, and create favorable conditions for unfriendly bacteria. You don't need to apply soap directly to your vulva; instead, you can simply wash it with warm water.

— **Decrease possible tissue irritation.** If you have vaginitis, use the methods we've covered in the previous pages to treat the condition as soon as it develops. Many women develop UTIs in conjunction with, or as a result of, vaginitis.

— **Manage your stress.** If you're under chronic stress, you become more vulnerable to many types of illness and infection, including UTIs. Women who have recurrent UTIs often become much less susceptible when they make lifestyle changes that reduce stress.

— **Use estrogen cream if you're menopausal.** Vaginal dryness, which you're most likely to experience in your 40s or later, also affects your urethral tissues and makes you more vulnerable to UTIs. By using a natural estrogen cream containing estriol, as recommended earlier in this chapter for VAD, you can enhance the integrity of your urethral tissues and help prevent UTIs.

Some women are more prone to UTIs than others. If you've made all the right lifestyle choices, but find that you still have a tendency to develop UTIs, drinking two or three cups of marsh-mallow root tea on a daily basis can soothe the tissues of your urethra and bladder and help prevent recurrent UTIs. To make the tea, add two tablespoons of marshmallow root to four cups of boil-ing water, simmer for 15 minutes, and strain.

If you tend to get UTIs after sex, you can also drink a half-teaspoon of D-mannose (available at most health-food stores), a natural sugar found in cranberries and pineapples, dissolved in a cup of water before or after you have sex. This helps eliminate unwanted bacteria from your urethra and bladder.

UTIs should always be treated as quickly as possible; if un-treated, they can soon lead to a kidney infection, which is a more serious condition, so antibiotics may be necessary. If you develop a UTI, you should have a urine test done by your naturopathic phy-sician or medical doctor. For a resource on treating UTIs naturally, see Appendix C.

Supporting Your Sexuality by Treating Interstitial Cystitis

Interstitial cystitis, a chronic inflammation of the bladder wall, is often misdiagnosed as a UTI or bladder infection. The symptoms can be similar: pain or burning sensations in the blad-der during or after urination, an urgency to urinate that may be intolerable, frequent urination, or pelvic pain. As with a UTI, the symptoms of interstitial cystitis can be intense, and treatment can radically improve your life—and your sex life. But unlike a UTI, with interstitial cystitis your urine test is normal and doesn't show any bacteria.

The cause of interstitial cystitis is unknown to Western medi-cine, but it may be due to disruption of the mucous membranes of the bladder, resulting from recurrent UTIs. Other causes may include environmental toxins, unidentified infections, autoimmune conditions, or (in some people) a defect in the bladder wall.

Like UTIs, interstitial cystitis is a predominantly female condition: nine out of ten people who have it are women. The condition can lead to chronic irritation of the bladder wall, and many women with interstitial cystitis have food sensitivities that provoke their symptoms.

If you have interstitial cystitis, your diagnosis will probably be made by an urologist who does an exam of your bladder wall, called a cystoscopy. Other tests may include a biopsy and a potassium chloride sensitivity test. The conventional treatment typically includes prescription drugs that affect the bladder wall, local medication, and pharmaceutical pain medications.

There are natural alternatives for treating interstitial cystitis and restoring the quality of your sex life without drugs. It's a complicated health issue that often calls for a multitiered solution, but with patience and perseverance you can reduce or eliminate the symptoms over time. You can begin treating interstitial cystitis by applying the following recommendations.

— **Soothe your bladder wall.** Drinking two or three cups of marshmallow root tea each day can mollify the mucous membranes of your bladder and urethra, and support the lining of your urinary tract. To make the tea, use the recipe recommended above for UTIs.

— **Remove irritating foods from your diet.** Avoiding foods that aggravate your symptoms, especially those that cause allergies and/or to which you are intolerant, is essential to treating interstitial cystitis. Your naturopathic doctor can order a blood test to determine these foods.

— **Support the lining of your bladder.** You can help restore your bladder lining by taking glucosamine sulfate as a dietary supplement. The recommended dose is 500 mg three times daily.

— **Maintain an alkaline-forming diet.** An alkaline-forming diet helps reduce the bladder pain of interstitial cystitis by keeping your urine alkaline. (See Appendix C for a resource on eating an alkaline-forming diet.) In addition, you can take 500 mg of calcium carbonate three times daily, or a quarter-teaspoon of baking soda twice daily.

— **Make sure you get adequate fluids.** By staying hydrated, you keep your urine diluted, which can reduce your symptoms; concentrated urine can irritate your bladder wall.

— **Prevent UTIs.** Interstitial cystitis makes you more vulnerable to urinary tract infections, which in turn can exacerbate your condition. Implement the measures recommended above for avoiding UTIs.

If you follow these recommendations consistently but your condition doesn't improve, see Appendix B to find a naturopathic doctor for further guidance. You may benefit from treatment with N-acetylglucosamine (NAG), which helps restore your bladder wall and decrease bladder pain. Homeopathic remedies, including cantharis, apis, and sarsasparilla, can treat painful urination and the urge to urinate. Physical therapy of your pelvic muscles, biofeedback, bladder retraining, diet therapy, stress reduction, and other techniques can reduce bladder pain and increase control over your bladder. If you're menopausal, your doctor may also recommend estriol cream or black-cohosh vaginal suppositories to support your tissues.

You may additionally benefit from traditional Chinese medicine, which treats interstitial cystitis by working with your chi. (Although Western medicine hasn't identified the underlying cause of the condition, in Chinese medicine it's seen as a chi imbalance.) Acupuncture and Chinese herbal medicines can decrease the pain associated with interstitial cystitis by stimulating the flow of chi through your pelvis and nourishing your yin and yang.

Enhancing Your Sexual Health
by Overcoming Ovarian Disorders

During your menstrual cycles your ovaries normally form small cysts, known as benign cysts because they're usually harmless and cause no symptoms. They often disappear on their own, but some may grow larger to the point that they compromise your health, as well as your sex life, and you need medical attention. An annual exam is recommended so your doctor can check for unusual cyst development; if any other ovarian mass is detected, a test will be done to rule out cancerous growth.

If you consistently develop benign cysts, they may cause sharp, intense pain during your ovulation. In this scenario, you'll most likely benefit from a hormone evaluation, which can help you prevent cysts by giving you information you need to balance your hormones. If you have frequent benign cysts, you also need to improve the circulation of blood and lymph in your pelvis. In addition, you can help prevent or treat cysts naturally, and boost the health of your ovaries at the same time, with the following.

— **Vitamins and diet.** Taking your daily multivitamin, eating foods containing vitamin A and beta-carotene, and adding flax and fish oils to your diet can all help prevent benign ovarian cysts.

— **Turska's formula**. A traditional Western herbal remedy, Turska's formula is an effective treatment for ovarian cysts. It isn't available as an over-the-counter product; you need to get a prescription from your naturopathic physician. (See Appendix B.)

— **Chinese herbal formulas.** By improving the flow of chi through your pelvis, Chinese herbal remedies can help prevent or treat ovarian cysts. A practitioner of Chinese medicine who specializes in herbal remedies can prepare a specific formula to match your unique symptoms.

— **Topical treatments.** Castor oil packs can help treat ovarian cysts by improving circulation of blood and lymph through your pelvis. See Appendix C for a resource on making castor oil packs.

Another ovarian challenge you may face is the condition known as polycystic ovarian syndrome, or PCOS. Many women have never heard of PCOS and have no idea what it is, but if you've experienced it you probably know its effects all too well. PCOS is linked with abnormal menstrual cycles, female infertility, weight gain, insulin resistance (a prediabetic condition), and other conditions, and may affect as many as 10 percent of women under age

45. Overcoming PCOS, as with frequent benign cysts, can greatly benefit sexuality and overall health.

In most cases, women with PCOS don't efficiently convert testosterone to estrogen in their bodies, resulting in an excess of testosterone. They often have irregular ovulation (or don't ovulate at all); an above-average number of ovarian cysts; or symptoms of hyperandrogenism, which may include head-hair loss, acne, or an increase of facial hair.

If you have PCOS, many natural treatments can help. Let's look at some of the most effective steps you can take to treat the condition.

— **Foods and dietary substances.** By including flax seeds, soy, and nettle root tea in your diet, you can increase your SHBG (sex hormone binding globulin), a protein that binds hormones so that you don't have too many active hormones in circulation. This helps reduce the elevated testosterone associated with PCOS.

— **Saw palmetto.** An herb often recommended to prevent male prostate enlargement, saw palmetto can be an effective treatment for women who have PCOS with symptoms of acne and hair loss. The recommended daily dose is 320 mg of a standardized extract of saw palmetto.

— **Spearmint tea.** Research shows that women with PCOS who drink a cup of spearmint tea twice daily for five days during the first two weeks of their menstrual cycles have a significant drop in their testosterone levels. They also have an increase in estrogen and other hormones that can help reverse PCOS.

— **Dietary and lifestyle changes.** If you have PCOS you can benefit from changes in your diet and lifestyle, especially if you also have insulin resistance. By combining a low-carbohydrate diet with an hour of aerobic exercise each day, you can significantly reduce some long-term effects of PCOS linked with insulin resistance, including diabetes and heart disease.

— **Chromium.** Dietary supplementation with this mineral can help decrease insulin resistance in women with PCOS, which in turn will make PCOS more manageable. The recommended daily dose is 500 mcg, but up to 2,000 mcg can be taken daily.

— **Acupuncture.** Research shows that acupuncture can benefit women with PCOS and infertility by helping to regulate their menstrual cycles and increasing their rate of pregnancies. If you have PCOS with infertility, see Appendix B for information on finding an acupuncturist.

Dispelling the Displeasure of Cervical Dysplasia

If you have cervical dysplasia, or abnormal changes in your cervical cells, it can be distressing, because cervical dysplasia is a potential precursor to cervical cancer. Some women with the condition undergo a surgical procedure known as *cervical conization,* which removes external tissue from the cervix. Despite this, the condition may return, and the procedure may be repeated multiple times to no avail. Cervical dysplasia can mean frequent visits to the doctor, many uncomfortable medical procedures, and lots of concern about spreading the virus that can cause the condition to your partner (he can become a carrier of the virus, which is contagious through sexual contact, and with some strains of it, he can get genital warts)—all of which can disrupt the quality of your sex life and compromise your experience of pleasure. For some women, cervical dysplasia might well be renamed *cervical displeasure.*

Cervical dysplasia is frequently caused by human papillomavirus, which is sexually transmitted. In addition to practicing safe sex (see Appendix G), you may be able to prevent cervical dysplasia, or heal your cervix if you have the condition, by keeping your immune system in top form. Preventing or treating cervical dysplasia can make a big difference in your sexual health, and one of the best ways to do so is by following the lifestyle, diet, and supplement recommendations in Chapter 2. You can also prevent or treat cervical dysplasia with the following:

— **Indole-3-carbinol.** Eat lots of cruciferous vegetables, which are high in indole-3-carbinol, or take 300 mg of indole-3-carbinol as a supplement daily. This helps lower your body's production of "unfriendly" estrogens, which in excess can stimulate estrogen receptors in your cervix and increase abnormal cell growth. Indole-3-carbinol also promotes "friendly" estrogens that don't increase the growth of abnormal cervical cells.

— **Folic acid.** An important B vitamin for cell reproduction, folic acid is helpful in preventing and treating abnormal growth of cervical cells. It can prevent abnormal cervical-cell changes from progressing, particularly in women who have been on birth-control pills. Most daily multivitamins contain 800 mcg of folic acid; for long-term prevention of abnormal cervical cells, take between 800 and 2,400 mcg daily.

— **Vitamin C.** To prevent abnormal cervical cell changes, take 2,000 mg daily; for treating the condition, take up to 6,000 mg daily for three months or more. (Note: Excessive vitamin C can cause diarrhea.)

— **Alpha lipoic acid.** To prevent abnormal cervical-cell changes, take 100 mg daily; for treatment, take up to 200 mg daily for three months or more.

— **Mixed carotenoids.** Mixed carotenoids combine alpha-carotene, beta-carotene, lutein, and other carotenoids. To prevent abnormal cervical-cell changes, take 50,000 IU daily; for treatment, take 150,000 IU daily for three months or more.

— **Chinese herbal formulas.** Supporting your immune system with Chinese herbs can balance your chi and help prevent or treat abnormal cervical-cell changes. A number of Chinese herbal formulas can also help restore cervical tissue that contains abnormal cells. A qualified practitioner of Chinese herbal medicine (see Appendix B) can prepare a formula suited to your personal needs.

— **Escharotic treatment.** Escharotic treatment is an herbal and nutritional therapy that has been used by naturopathic doctors for many years to treat women with abnormal cervical cells, as well as to prevent recurrences of the condition. Therapy typically consists of weekly treatments for three to five weeks, depending on the degree of abnormal cell growth and other factors. To

89

determine if escharotic treatment is appropriate for you, consult a licensed naturopathic physician. (See Appendix B.)

Beyond Pelvic Pain—and into Pelvic Pleasure

A number of conditions categorized under the general term *pelvic pain* can interfere with your ability to enjoy sex. Pelvic pain can be experienced in your vulva, your vagina, or elsewhere in your pelvis. It can be caused by many factors, and some types of pelvic pain can be a challenge to diagnose and treat. If you suffer from the condition, solving it can transform your sex life; getting past pelvic pain unburdens your libido, freeing it up to replace the pangs of pain with welcome waves of well-being.

You may have experienced acute pelvic pain—for example, if your partner's penis makes sudden contact with your cervix during sex. But pelvic pain can also be chronic; if you have a history of pelvic surgery, or if you've had a difficult labor, you may be prone to a chronically tight, shortened PC muscle, resulting in pain with intercourse. Other conditions associated with pelvic pain include *vulvodynia* (chronic pain at the vulva), *vulvovestibulitis* (chronic inflammation of the vulva and vaginal opening), and *vaginismus* (painful spasms and contractions in the vagina).

The topic of pelvic pain can involve complex issues that go beyond the reach of this chapter; there are numerous resources, as well as support groups, for women suffering from these conditions. However, if you experience pelvic pain, especially vulvar pain, there's one method of treatment you should know about—a unique do-it-yourself approach that can be highly effective, and that too few women are aware of, known as vaginal steam baths. Not only can this method relieve or cure pelvic pain, but it's also a soothing, nourishing way to connect with your sexuality and femininity.

Vaginal steam baths, which have been used traditionally in Korea and parts of South America, provide you with numerous other potential benefits. They can help decrease skin inflammation if you have a vulvar yeast infection, and help heal your tissues if you've had an episiotomy, vulvar biopsy, or other surgical procedure in or near your vulva. They can also loosen and relax your PC muscle, promote increased circulation, and may allow for easier penetration with intercourse if you have a condition associated with pelvic pain.

Vaginal steam baths are easy to do, and you can make each bath different by including various herbs or essential oils for added benefits. To get started, boil four cups of filtered water and pour it into a large stainless-steel or glass bowl. Add any herbs or essential oils you'd like to use, as described below, then place the bowl beneath a patio chair, or other type of chair with openings or slats in the seat, so you can sit with your naked vulva exposed to the steam. (Vaginal steam baths might be more aptly named *vulvar steam baths,* since the steam doesn't reach your vagina, which is internal.) Alternatively, you can place the bowl in a toilet, after turning off the toilet's water source and flushing to empty the water.

Before exposing your delicate vulvar tissues to the steam, test it carefully with your inner wrist so you won't burn yourself. Once you've established a comfortable temperature, stay seated in your steam bath, allowing your vulva and entire pelvis to relax, for about 15 minutes or until the steam subsides. For treating most kinds of pelvic pain, it's recommended that you do steam baths at least once a day for a week, and continue as needed to relieve your symptoms. To provide extra healing benefits, you can add the following herbs and essential oils, alone or in combination, to your steam baths:

— **Red clover.** This plant has been used in Western herbal medicine for decades to strengthen and tone the pelvic organs and tissues; it's often recommended to help prepare the uterus for childbirth. Sprinkle one teaspoon of dried or fresh red clover into your steam bath.

— **Oregano and tea-tree oil combined.** To relieve pelvic pain and itching related to a vulvar yeast infection, add one teaspoon of dried oregano, or one drop of oregano oil, and two drops of tea-tree oil to your steam bath. Both of these herbs have potent antifungal properties. (For a vulvar yeast infection, steam at least twice daily.)

— **Rose essential oil.** To alleviate vulvar discomfort and moisten your skin and tissues, add three drops of this essential oil to your steam bath. Rose essential oil is also used in aromatherapy to treat physical and emotional imbalances. Physically, it's recommended for low libido, infertility, and heavy menstrual bleeding. On an emotional level, it's recommended as a calming and harmonizing agent, and also as a catalyst to create an atmosphere of safety for bringing feelings about sexuality and self-esteem to the surface.

— **Lavender essential oil.** An anti-inflammatory that promotes tissue healing, this essential oil is also used in aromatherapy to promote both physical health (especially for your skin) and emotional harmony (to induce calmness, relieve nervous tension, and support your capacity for love and appreciation of beauty). To enhance your steam bath with lavender's healing effects, add three drops of lavender essential oil.

— **Rose and lavender essential oils combined.** Adding three drops of each of these essential oils to your steam bath can have a synergistic effect that's especially helpful in treating vulvar pain. (Even if you don't have pain, this treatment is recommended as a nurturing experience for this sensitive part of your body, particularly if you feel emotionally disconnected from your pelvis and sexuality.)

— **Red clover, lavender, calendula, and chamomile combined.** To relieve and gently heal any vulvar inflammation or dryness, add one teaspoon of each of these herbs, as either dried or fresh flowers, to your steam bath. Along with the benefits of red clover outlined above, lavender, calendula, and chamomile all have anti-inflammatory and soothing effects on the delicate tissues of your vulva (and they also make a beautiful floating bouquet).

Conclusion: The Culmination of Your Sexual-Core Health

In this chapter, we've delved into the fabulous anatomy of your pelvis—the diverse, dynamic region of your body that allows you to experience sex, reach orgasm, menstruate, release eggs, grow a fetus, and more. You've discovered exercises and other tools for strengthening your sexual core, enhancing the health of your phenomenal feminine organs, and maximizing your many-splendored potential for pleasure. You've also discovered natural, sex-boosting solutions to common challenges that you may encounter in this most vital area of your body.

As you've seen throughout this chapter, not only does your pelvis play a pivotal role in your capacity for pleasure, but it's also the nucleus of your chi and central to your overall health. Now that we've explored the keys for optimizing the health of your sexual core, we're ready to begin a new passage in our journey. In the next chapter, we'll explore the rich realm of your hormones, and all that you can do to boost your libido and well-being by enhancing your hormonal health. As we move forward, the tools and insights you've discovered thus far will merge with many other discoveries you'll make.

CHAPTER 4

HARMONIZING YOUR HORMONES

Sex in the Balance

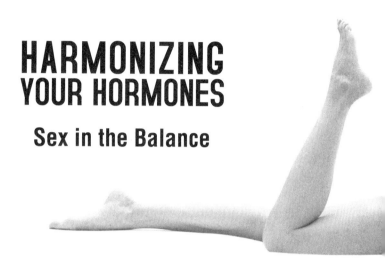

"Our bodies act as incredibly accurate barometers that indicate how closely we live our lives in-line with our true heart's desires."

— CHRISTIANE NORTHRUP, M.D., *THE SECRET PLEASURES OF MENOPAUSE*

Your magnificent hormones drift through your body, profoundly affecting who you are, how you feel, and your overall health and vitality. They constantly influence your thoughts, emotions, behavior, and spirit, often exerting a powerful pull on even your most subtle urges and inclinations. In fact, the word *hormone* derives from *hormé,* Greek for "impulse."

Perhaps more than anything else, your hormones affect your sexuality, intimately shaping your experiences of love, attraction, and arousal. (*Hormone* is also related to the Greek *ornynai,* which means "to rouse.") If there's one thing you can do to enhance the quality of your sexuality, stay healthy, and keep your zest for life, it's to create and maintain your hormonal balance.

Your hormones are not only an integral part of your personality, but also an extraordinary physiological phenomenon—tiny biologically active substances that are released by your glands, circulate in your body fluids, and have strong effects on parts of your anatomy far from their points of origin. Every day, a choreographed dance takes place within your physical self as these complex, multifaceted substances intermingle to create your unique sexual nature. The intricacies of this dance extend even beyond your body; your hormones ultimately connect you with your environment, inviting you to join with another who can share your passions and pleasures, bond with you, and join you in the dance.

As you go through your life, this choreography passes through many delicate transitions—hormones stimulate the changes of puberty, ovulation, menstruation, fertility, pregnancy, perimenopause, menopause, and postmenopause—and a new kind of hormonal harmony gradually emerges during every phase. Each new dance of your sexual health is as elaborate as anything you've previously experienced and perhaps even more extraordinary. Even as you pass through new transformations, your hormones continue to move in elegant synchronized patterns, your sexual nature gently re-creates itself, and the dance goes on.

In this chapter, you'll learn about the important and remarkably resilient role your hormones play in your sexuality and health, and many ways you can nurture and preserve their equilibrium through all of your hormonal transitions. You'll discover which of your hormones you most need to know about to support your sexuality, which are most likely to be out of balance during certain phases of your life, and the essential natural tools you need to correct those imbalances and enhance your libido—including herbal remedies, nutritional support, bioidentical hormones, and more.

Your Six Key Hormones: The Great Sex Sextet

In order to harmonize your hormones and enhance your sexuality, you would do well to become acquainted with the key players in the dance—the chemical messengers that moisten, relax, nourish, empower, energize, revitalize, and sensualize you on a daily basis. Their names are familiar: *estrogen, progesterone, DHEA, testosterone, cortisol,* and *thyroid hormone.* You have other hormones in your body as well, but we call these six the Great Sex Sextet because of the important roles they play in your sexuality. When they're each in balance, you tend to feel like your healthiest self, capable of practically anything you put your mind to, and fully able to manifest your sexual energy; if they aren't in balance, you feel robbed of your potential, both sexually and otherwise.

In the pages ahead, as we explore each of these hormones, we'll focus primarily on how each affects your body, mind, and sexuality from the perspective of Western medicine. We'll also touch on the nature of hormones from the standpoint of Chinese medicine—their "energetic" qualities, typically overlooked in the West. As you've discovered, Chinese medicine teaches that your chi consists of yin and yang energy: yin is inward, contractive, relaxing, moistening, and feminine; and yang is outward, expansive, stimulating, drying, and masculine. As a practitioner trained in both Western science and Chinese medicine, I've found that some hormones tend to be more yin, and others more yang, in their effects on your body.

Each hormone in your Great Sex Sextet has a unique place on the yin–yang continuum: Estrogen is the most yin, followed by progesterone, which is mainly yin but with some yang actions, and DHEA is less yin than progesterone. Continuing in ascending order of yang energy, you have testosterone, followed by cortisol, with thyroid hormone being the most yang.

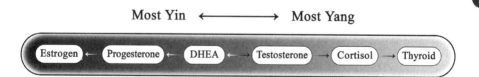

The yin and yang properties of your hormones can also be illustrated with the familiar yin/yang symbol, although it's important to note that some hormones—particularly progesterone and DHEA—can have both yin and yang effects on your body.

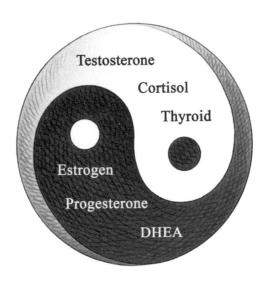

As long as all of these hormones work well together, you'll have hormonal harmony and sexual health. To experience full sexual arousal, you need to be contractive and relaxed (yin), but you also need to be expansive and stimulated (yang). Let's take a look at each of the hormones on your yin–yang continuum, and how they influence your sexuality.

Estrogen: Your Compassion (and Passion) Hormone

Estrogen is your great connector; it enhances your feelings of intimacy and tenderness, and facilitates your ability to bond deeply with another person. Essential to your sexuality, it sustains and promotes your femininity, keeping your libido primed to flow in abundance. Estrogen is also life giving; when you were in your mother's womb, you were bathed in a protective layer of uterine tissue that was stimulated to develop by estrogen.

From the Chinese medicine perspective, estrogen is important to your vitality, and very yin because it softens, moistens, nurtures, allows for greater flexibility, and accentuates your deepest feminine nature. As you'll discover, it's because of fluctuations in your estrogen level that your body releases your "Heavenly Water" during much of your life.

At puberty, a surge of estrogen fleshed out your hips, breasts, and curves, and developed body hair in your most intimate places, as you magically blossomed into a young woman. Each month during your menstruating years, estrogen enhances your fertility and forms the lining in your uterus—the endometrium—to cushion and support a potential embryo. If pregnancy doesn't take place, as your estrogen level drops, the lining sloughs off and becomes your menstrual flow.

Through your menstrual cycles, estrogen connects you with the phases of the moon. For many women, the monthly rise and fall of estrogen creates cycles that closely correspond to the lunar calendar. Ancient cultures recognized this link between menstrual cycles and the natural world: the words *month, moon,* and *menstrual* all share a common ancestral root.

Estrogen, which is made in your ovaries and adrenal glands, is critical for your sexual energy and vitality in many ways. One of the most important is its ability to support your libido by interacting with testosterone in your brain. You need adequate amounts of both estrogen and testosterone to turn on your brain's arousal circuits. When you have optimal estrogen, testosterone can effectively stimulate nerve receptors to create the sparks that kindle passion and pleasure.

Estrogen can help you feel good in other ways as well. It's directly linked with your sense of well-being, because it works with serotonin (your "feel-good" brain chemical) to enhance your moods. Serotonin increases feelings of happiness and decreases feelings of anxiety, and research shows that estrogen and serotonin levels rise and fall in tandem. This is why many women have mood swings, feel depressed, and experience erratic food cravings before their periods, but not at other times in their cycles.

As you discovered in Chapter 3, estrogen plays a key role in your potential for sexual pleasure by maintaining the health and elasticity of your vaginal and vulvar tissues, including your clitoris, urethra, and inner and outer labia. These tissues are estrogen-dependent, which means they need adequate estrogen to stay flexible and moist. Without sufficient estrogen, they can lose much of their natural lubrication, making pleasurable sex difficult or impossible. (Estrogen also supports connective tissues throughout your body—it can serve as a natural moisturizer; improve collagen content; help prevent wrinkles; and give you soft, smooth, supple skin.) And as you've also seen, estrogen helps maintain the ideal pH of your vaginal tissues, thwarting vaginal infections due to bacteria or yeast, as well as urinary tract infections—either of which can obstruct your enjoyment of sex.

Estrogen not only played a major role in enlarging your breasts at puberty—like fertilizer to soil, it allowed them to bloom from tiny buds to the fuller breasts of a woman—but during each of your menstrual cycles, as your estrogen levels wax and wane, so does the volume of your breast tissue. Estrogen also heightens the touch-sensitivity of your breasts, which are important for your femininity, integral to your sensual arousal and response, and attractive to your partner.

Other benefits of estrogen include increasing your stress tolerance, preventing inflammation in your brain, potentially helping to maintain your memory, and supporting your blood-brain barrier—a thin cover that protects your brain from environmental insults and toxins. Researchers hypothesize that women may help preserve their brain cells and prevent age-related dementia if they begin taking estrogen in early menopause.[1]

Your bones thrive in the presence of estrogen. This hormone stimulates cells that build new bone, and inhibits ones that pull calcium from your bones. Having adequate levels of estrogen from your teens to your 40s is important for maintaining healthy, strong bones; it helps you make deposits into your "bone bank"— which you need when your hormone levels and bone density drop at menopause.

Estrogen is your best friend when you have just the right amount, but a foe if you have too much or too little. An excess can lead to breast cysts, heavy menstrual cycles, exaggerated premenstrual symptoms, uterine fibroid tumors, and ovarian cysts, as well as increase your risk of estrogen-related cancers. Insufficient estrogen can cause you to feel irritable and overwhelmed;

---

[1] A note on our use of the term *menopause:* Although menopause is typically defined as the year that begins with your last period, for the purposes of this chapter we often use the term to include perimenopause, the period of time leading up to menopause, during which you begin to experience midlife hormonal changes like irregular menstrual cycles.

result in the discomforts some women experience postpartum; and lead to menopausal symptoms of insomnia, anxiety, hot flashes, and vaginal dryness. Later in this chapter, you'll discover different kinds of estrogen, ways of enhancing your body's ability to produce the friendliest forms, and how to use natural bioidentical estrogen replacement.

Taking Care of Your Breasts

The health of your breasts is a part of your sexual health, and reflective of your overall wellness. All of the lifestyle tips you've explored earlier in this book will help you maintain healthy breasts. To further preserve your breast health, be aware of your risk factors for breast cancer, examine your breasts often, and get screened regularly for cancer. Remember that your breasts are more highly hormone-sensitive than other parts of your body. Use hormone replacement therapy only if you have to, and take the lowest dose you can for the shortest time necessary. If you take estrogen or progesterone for menopausal symptoms, use only natural, bioidentical hormones.

Progesterone: Your Libido-Grounding Hormone

Progesterone helps maintain your hormonal equilibrium and provide a strong, stable basis for your libido. In addition, it can ease anxiety, induce restful sleep, and "relax" your connective tissues. It has primarily yin qualities, but can also be yang in its support of your energy-building adrenal glands.

Made in your ovaries and adrenal glands, progesterone has a unique ability to enhance your sexuality because it can be a precursor to testosterone—as you'll discover, your sexiest hormone—and promote your body's production of cortisol, which can also affect your libido. In addition, progesterone influences your sexual energy by supporting your thyroid hormone (which regulates the metabolism of every cell in your body), and nurtures your libido by helping you sleep. Being able to sleep soundly can increase your ability to take pleasure in sex . . . to sleep, perchance to enhance.

When progesterone is released after you ovulate, it helps prevent estrogen from becoming too prolific, and your uterine lining from becoming too thick. It can also help settle down your nervous system and reduce heart palpitations associated with menopausal hormone changes.

If you're in your middle or late 30s and you want to become pregnant, taking natural progesterone may improve your fertility by helping prepare your uterine lining for a fertilized egg to implant. Many patients in this age bracket who try unsuccessfully to become pregnant for many months, or years, easily conceive once they start taking natural progesterone.

If you become pregnant, your levels of progesterone soar in support of your pregnancy, with many effects and benefits. You may have a "pregnancy glow," and the feelings of well-being and vibrant health that many women describe when pregnant; both can be due, in part, to progesterone. By relaxing your connective tissues, the surge of progesterone helps soften your ligaments and allow for the baby's safe passage through your pelvis.

Progesterone can also come to your aid if you experience postpartum depression. After childbirth your hormone levels, including progesterone, decline sharply. Taking natural progesterone can mitigate feelings of despair during this otherwise special time.

Like many women, you may experience decreasing levels of progesterone in your late 30s or early 40s. This can be the result of a stressful lifestyle or simply because you're entering a less fertile time in your life. Either way, you may tend to have an imbalance—not enough progesterone compared to estrogen—creating a condition called *estrogen dominance*. Symptoms include increased breast tenderness, breast swelling, water retention in your tissues, bloating (especially of the abdomen), increased premenstrual symptoms, exacerbated menstrual cramps, heavier periods, and more clotting in your menstrual flow.

A classic sign that you may have inadequate progesterone is insomnia in the second half of your menstrual cycle—particularly if you often awaken in the middle of the night and can't get back to sleep. Another sign is anxiety that occurs only during the second half of your cycle; progesterone has the ability to activate GABA receptors in your brain that induce mental calmness. Both of these symptoms can compromise your libido, since adequate sleep and a calm mind are essential for your peak sexual energy.

Many symptoms of low progesterone can be alleviated with herbal support to enhance your body's natural progesterone production or by taking natural bioidentical progesterone in the second half of your cycle. As you continue this chapter, you'll discover more about both approaches.

Your Moon Cycle:
The Ebb and Flow of Your "Heavenly Water"

If you're the typical female, your "moon cycle" begins around age 12 and continues until about age 50, when you experience a gradual cessation of your cycles. Day one of your cycle is the first day of your period; the initial part of your 28-day cycle, typically the first 14 days, is known as the *follicular phase*. During this phase, estrogen predominates, reaching its highest level and stimulating the growth of your uterine lining. If you have regular menstrual cycles, you're most likely to be fertile at midcycle, around day 14, when you ovulate (release a ripe egg) and your ovaries form a tissue mass called the *corpus luteum,* which releases progesterone. Your sexual appetite crests during the follicular phase, becoming especially yang at midcycle, when your urge to procreate is strongest.

During the second half of your cycle, known as the *luteal phase,* progesterone is abundant, and estrogen is also likely to be high. At the end of your cycle, estrogen and progesterone both plummet, allowing your body to release the endometrial lining as your menstrual flow, and your sexual energy wanes.

Traditional Chinese medicine provides a refreshing alternative to modern terms like *menstrual flow* or the generic *period.* As mentioned in the Introduction to this book, ancient Chinese practitioners didn't refer to a woman's menstrual flow as blood, but rather as her "Heavenly Water." (It was sometimes also called her "Dew of Heaven.") Like many women in the West, you may feel that the topic of menstruation is saturated with negative connotations. Imagine how differently you might feel about your monthly flow if you consistently described it with such a heavenly metaphor!

DHEA: Your Sexy Hormone

A hormone with far-reaching effects, DHEA (short for the tongue twister *dehydroepiandrosterone*) elevates your libido, induces a sense of well-being, enhances fertility, builds bones, and more. With both yin and yang qualities, it nourishes your brain and ovaries while also supporting your entire hormonal system, especially your adrenal glands, and building your overall health.

DHEA is produced primarily by your adrenal glands, but also by your ovaries and brain. It enhances your sexuality; and sex, in turn, can increase its release in your body. Some of the health benefits of sex that we outlined at the beginning of Chapter 1 are due, in part, to the release of DHEA during arousal and orgasm.

DHEA's ability to boost your libido and your moods was demonstrated in a study published in 2005 in the *Archives of General Psychiatry,* which found that supplemental DHEA significantly improved sexual functioning and successfully treated depression in women and men aged 45 to 65. Although the dose was unusually high, it powerfully impacted the libido and mental state of those who took it. Another study, which showed that DHEA can enhance fertility and pregnancy rates in older women (by increasing the quality of their eggs), confirmed its beneficial effects on sex and mood; a number of the study's participants reported "side effects" of increased libido and improved well-being.

The secret to DHEA's ability to enhance your sexuality is biochemical: as a precursor to testosterone, it plays a pivotal role in your "hormone cascade." The diagram below shows how pregnenolone, your "mother" hormone, is a precursor to many of your other important hormones, and how they all interact in your body.

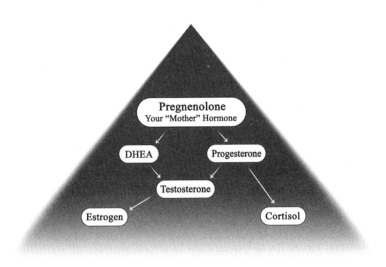

Your hormone cascade.

As you can see, DHEA converts directly into testosterone, and via testosterone, into estrogen—which is why many women need only tiny amounts of DHEA to experience dramatic libido-enhancing effects, particularly during and after midlife. DHEA is most effective when other hormones, especially estrogen, are well balanced, and it seems especially beneficial for women who are overstressed and need to rejuvenate their bodies, minds, and spirits.

While DHEA is busy enhancing your sexuality, it's also giving you other noteworthy benefits that indirectly support your libido-building lifestyle. Studies show it can improve memory and concentration, and by stimulating cells that lay down new bone tissue, improve female bone density—which can be especially important for menopausal women.

If your DHEA level is low, you're likely to experience reduced libido, a diminished sense of well-being, and lower overall vitality. Other symptoms may include fatigue, decreased memory, reduced fertility, poorer bone and adrenal-gland health, and a general reduction in your hormonal health. As you move forward in this chapter, you'll discover how to evaluate your DHEA level and, if it's low, use natural bioidentical DHEA to correct your symptoms. DHEA is best used under the guidance of a skilled health-care professional; an excessive amount can have effects in your body similar to those induced by androgens (male sex hormones), such as acne, increased facial hair, balding, and anxiety.

Testosterone: Your Even Sexier Hormone

You may think of testosterone as the male sex hormone, but it's very much *your* hormone, too. Produced naturally by your ovaries and adrenal glands, it's vital to your sexuality and health. Not only do you need it for a healthy libido, but it also energizes your entire being and helps keep you "jazzed" about your life. Testosterone is mostly yang—exciting; uplifting; and with qualities that allow for growth, outward motion, and creativity—and it can supercharge your sexual chi, which has powerful healing potential for your body, mind, and spirit.

As we touched on earlier in this chapter, testosterone, with the assistance of estrogen, stimulates nerve receptors in your brain, igniting your pleasure circuitry and setting sexual feelings and arousal in motion. At the same time, testosterone can give an added jolt to your sexuality by increasing your clitoris's sensitivity to touch.

Testosterone can have wide-ranging effects on your personality, giving you an extra "edge" that may be felt in your sexual energy, or anywhere else in your life. For example, it may help you become more assertive, develop a take-charge attitude, maintain your dynamic creative drive, or summon the confidence to hold firm boundaries when you need to.

Like DHEA, testosterone can also increase your sense of well-being. Research has shown that testosterone plays a role in modulating the actions of dopamine—a brain chemical that allows you to feel joy and pleasure. When women have deficient dopamine, they're subject not only to reduced sex drive but also feelings of hopelessness and decreased ability to handle stress.

Testosterone gives you additional benefits not directly connected to your sexuality: It helps build your bones and prevent bone loss, maintain a balanced ratio of fat to lean muscle mass, and improve your muscle strength. During midlife, it can help reduce hot flashes, night sweats, and headaches. Testosterone can also help protect your brain cells from injury, and research shows that it may help prevent the "tangled-up" neurons in the brain associated with Alzheimer's disease.

You need a sufficient amount of testosterone in your body to make all of its benefits possible. If your level is too low, in addition to experiencing diminished libido and feeling lackluster about sex, you're apt to be uninterested in trying new activities and feel "drab," worn-out, and tired much of the time.

Many women who take natural testosterone find that it stimulates both their sensuality and their senses. Along with resurrected sexual desire, they often describe feeling as if they're having flashbacks to how they felt at earlier times in their lives when healthy levels of hormones coursed through their bodies—more alert and alive than they've felt in years, more perceptive, and more attuned to new sensations and their environment. Some say they feel their awareness reawakening, after long slumber, to all the possibilities inherent in their bodies.

It appears that in some situations testosterone can reduce risk of breast cancer. A study reported in *Breast Cancer Research* in 2009 found that when women take bioidentical hormone therapy such as estrogen and progesterone, taking testosterone as part of the regimen may decrease breast-cancer risk. This may be due to several mechanisms of testosterone, including its abilities to increase cancer-cell death and to change receptors on estrogen-sensitive cells (which are otherwise more cancer-prone with estrogen therapy).

Later in this chapter, you'll discover more about testosterone, including the natural bioidentical testosterone prescription that's best for many women.

Your Hormones and Your Jing

Practitioners of ancient Chinese medicine couldn't isolate hormones and examine them with microscopes, and they had no concept of hormones as we know them. But through careful observation they understood their energetic actions and effects on a woman's sexuality during every phase of her life.

The traditional Chinese notion that perhaps comes closest to reflecting our modern Western understanding of hormones is *jing*— a form of your chi passed down to you by your ancestors, and a part of your life beginning with your conception. The effects of abundant jing in your body can be much like the effects of healthy, balanced hormones in Western medicine.

If you spend your jing carefully, you increase your chances of living to a healthy, ripe old age. You can preserve your jing with a life of moderation, eating good food, getting adequate sleep, and nourishing your body. You can also recycle your jing and strengthen it with certain techniques and sexual practices, some of which we'll explore later in this book. In terms of your sexuality, if you have abundant jing, you have the energy and vitality to enjoy a robust sex life.

On the other hand, if you spend your jing quickly, you're more prone to illness and low energy, including diminished sexual energy. You can exhaust your jing with a high-stress life; a poor diet; inadequate sleep; and excessive prescription or recreational drugs, smoking, or alcohol.

Cortisol: Your Stimulating Hormone

Produced in the small adrenal glands that sit atop your kidneys, cortisol is the "stress hormone" your body releases when you feel as if you're running behind schedule, under pressure, and racing to catch up. Your adrenal glands are surprisingly important for your sexuality; cortisol is a stimulating, yang hormone that can make or break your libido. Let's take a closer look at your critical cortisol-sex connection.

With cortisol, balance is everything. If you don't have enough, your libido suffers, you tend to feel tired all the time, you lack your get-up-and-go, and your immune system doesn't work optimally. But if your cortisol is consistently too high, day after day, as a result of chronic stress in your life, your libido is also likely to crash, in part because constant stress is exhausting and depletes the energy you need to be sexually responsive. Too much cortisol also results in feelings of fragility and agitation—not exactly what you need for great sex—and causes you to gain weight, especially around your waist.

Excessive cortisol can wreak hormonal havoc by throwing your other hormones out of balance and jeopardizing many of the benefits they offer for your sexuality and health. Instead of consistent menstrual cycles with balanced levels of estrogen, progesterone, DHEA, and testosterone, your body may experience a continuous "alarm" state. As a result, you may not ovulate, which lowers your progesterone level and in turn can cause much heavier menstrual flow and worsened PMS symptoms—again, hardly what you want to put you in the mood for pleasure. In addition, excessive cortisol can inhibit the function of your thyroid hormone, which, as you'll discover, also contributes to your libido.

When you have the right level of cortisol, it benefits your health and sexual energy in myriad ways. It gives you the opportunity to fully experience your libido, supports the health of your immune system, and promotes normal blood-sugar regulation. If you have stress in your life, it helps you respond in an appropriate, healthy way.

Your body has a natural cortisol rhythm that also supports your health and sexuality. You feel best when your level is high in the morning and slowly subsides toward evening; you get out of bed bursting with energy, and at the end of the day you feel tired and readily able to fall asleep. Paradoxically, cortisol is a stress hormone that helps you sleep through the night. A healthy cortisol level provides energy you need by day, yet quiets your mind at night, allowing your body to rejuvenate, heal from illness, and maintain a healthy libido.

If your natural cycle of cortisol is out of kilter—as a result of unmitigated stress or low blood sugar—your cortisol level may be low in the morning and high at night. In this scenario, you can experience difficulty waking in the morning, and insomnia at night—a major libido killer.

When you're asleep, cortisol is responsible for converting sugar into glucose to feed your sleeping brain. You need a steady supply of glucose, throughout the night, to get a full night's rest, but if your cortisol is too low, you don't convert enough glucose to let your brain stay asleep through the night. At some point your brain gets "starved" of glucose, and your adrenal glands start sending out adrenaline, another stress hormone, instead of cortisol. You may experience what amounts to an adrenaline rush in the middle of the night, waking suddenly, as if an alarm has gone off in your head, with your thoughts racing. It may be hours before you can fall back to sleep.

Many people are unaware that insufficient cortisol at night can be caused by past lifestyle issues. For instance, if in the past you've had chronically high cortisol that resulted from unrelenting stress, your adrenal glands can become "burned-out" and unable to release adequate cortisol when you need it. You can remain in that state long after the period of stress has passed.

Another cortisol imbalance that can deplete your sexual energy, also caused by chronic stress, is known as *cortisol steal*. This happens when a high demand for cortisol "steals" from your production of other hormones. As you saw in the "hormone cascade" diagram earlier in this chapter, your hormones are interrelated, and some can be converted into others. If you have a typical case of cortisol steal, your body responds to the cortisol demand by converting some of your progesterone into cortisol; as a result, your progesterone isn't able to perform all of its important functions. Cortisol essentially pilfers progesterone, your progesterone gets shortchanged, and your health and libido suffer the consequences.

In an extreme case of cortisol steal, one of my patients survived a frightening near-death experience, after which she remained for years in a state of post-traumatic stress that exhausted her adrenal glands and caused acutely imbalanced hormone levels. Although only in her 30s, she stopped menstruating, her hair turned white, and she effectively went into early menopause. In an effort to meet the urgent demand for cortisol, her body had "stolen" from its production of estrogen, progesterone, DHEA, and testosterone. (Fortunately, she was able to recover, and eventually resumed having periods.) This shows what can happen in a woman's body under unusual stress, but even low stress, on a daily basis, can gradually increase your body's cortisol demand to the point that your overall hormone production becomes imbalanced. This can have far-reaching effects on your hormonal health, wear down your body, and deprive you of many of the joys of a healthy sex life.

If you're chronically stressed as you approach midlife, and your cortisol is in high demand and your adrenal glands can't keep up with your body's other hormonal needs—particularly if you're ovulating inconsistently, or not at all—you may experience an especially difficult menopausal transition. When your ovaries go through their natural midlife "career change" and stop producing hormones, your adrenal glands normally pick up where your ovaries leave off. But if chronic stress has compromised your adrenal glands, they have a hard time stepping up to the plate. This can result in exaggerated menopausal symptoms: excessive insomnia, dramatic night sweats and hot flashes, and erratic mood changes. Healthy adrenal-gland function and cortisol production are essential to a strong menopausal transition and a vigorous midlife libido.

As you continue with this chapter, you'll discover how you can keep your cortisol-producing adrenal glands strong and vital, and also support your sexuality and health, with dietary tips, herbs, nutritional supplements, and natural bioidentical hormones.

Thyroid: Your Power Hormone

You may have noticed that thyroid hormone isn't on the "hormone cascade" diagram. Unlike the other hormones we've explored, it doesn't come from pregnenolone. It's made in your thyroid gland, a dynamic butterfly-shaped organ just below your Adam's apple. A powerhouse for energy production in your body, your thyroid gland is essential for your libido, and the hormone it releases is very yang in its ability to generate your sexual energy.

Most people, although not all, naturally tend toward a healthy thyroid-hormone level. By following the lifestyle recommendations previously outlined in this book—and especially by managing stress—you increase your chances of maintaining one. You may not be aware of all the benefits that stem from having your thyroid hormone at a healthy level, but you're apt to feel them everywhere in your life—including your sex life. Your thyroid hormone helps create the energy you need to forge through challenging situations, overcome barriers, achieve your dreams, maximize your health . . . and have great sex.

Your level of thyroid hormone is vital to your capacity for pleasure because too much or too little can send your sexuality and your health into a tailspin. If you have too much, a condition known as *hyperthyroidism,* you can have an increased heart rate, anxiety, or weight loss. If you have insufficient thyroid hormone, or *hypothyroidism*—a far more common condition among women—it can slow your entire metabolism and cause a host of symptoms, including decreased interest in sex, difficulty responding to sexual stimulation, and problems achieving orgasm. Restoring your thyroid hormone can be one of the most important steps you take to enhance your sexual responsiveness, orgasmic potential, and quality of life.

In addition to decreased sex drive, your symptoms if you have low thyroid hormone may include irregular or heavy menstrual cycles, PMS, excessive fatigue, sluggishness, depression, easy weight gain, insomnia, headaches, migraines, digestive problems, and constipation. Having low thyroid hormone reduces your body temperature, so the condition can also cause an aversion to cold weather, chronically cold hands and feet, and poor circulation. If you have low thyroid hormone in midlife, you're prone to severe menopausal symptoms, including vaginal dryness that doesn't fully respond to topical estrogen.

Since low thyroid hormone reduces the rate of your metabolism, it can cause other symptoms that affect organs and systems throughout your body. If you have the condition, you probably won't have all of these symptoms, but you may recognize some of them: heart palpitations, an inability to lose weight, high cholesterol, low blood sugar, decreased immunity, difficulty getting up in the morning, puffiness in your face and eyelids when you wake, joint and muscle pain, dry skin and hair, hair loss (including a tendency to lose the outer third of your eyebrows), infertility, recurrent miscarriages, anxiety, hives, and allergies.

If you have low thyroid hormone, it can be difficult for a doctor to diagnose accurately. Laboratory tests aren't always definitive, borderline cases are often overlooked, and you can have low thyroid hormone even if your test says you're normal—a condition known as "subclinically low" thyroid. Yet if you have low thyroid hormone, you may suffer needlessly, for years, from many of the above symptoms.

Understanding how your thyroid hormone works can be helpful if you need to restore it to a healthy level. Although we refer to "thyroid hormone" in the singular, you actually have more than one thyroid hormone. One of them, known as *thyroid stimulating hormone,* or TSH, is what's usually tested to find out whether you have low thyroid hormone. (In the pages ahead, and in Appendix E, we'll look more closely at thyroid-hormone evaluation and testing.) TSH stimulates your thyroid gland to release an inactive thyroid hormone called *T4,* which your liver converts into an active thyroid hormone known as *T3.* You want to have a healthy level of active T3, because it stimulates all of your cells to make energy, both sexual and otherwise.

One cause of low thyroid hormone is stress that won't go away. If you're under incessant stress, imbalanced cortisol can impede your ability to convert T4 into active T3; instead, it's converted into an inactive form called *Reverse T3.* Without enough T3, you may stop ovulating, which in turn can cause many hormone imbalances, including estrogen dominance—too much estrogen compared to progesterone. In a vicious cycle, this can be detrimental to your thyroid-hormone function. (On the other hand, when you have a healthy thyroid-hormone level and you ovulate regularly, you release progesterone on schedule, and, in a virtuous cycle, this supports your thyroid-hormone function.)

As we move forward, you'll discover natural remedies you can use to treat thyroid imbalances and help keep your thyroid hormone at a healthy, libido-supporting level.

Evaluating Your Hormones:
How "Hormonious" Are You?

Now that we've delved into the nature of each of the six hormones that make up your Great Sex Sextet, let's look at the most useful tests you can use to gauge their status in your body. As you've seen, you need adequate levels of each of these hormones to experience peak sexual arousal and optimal health.

Evaluating the key players in your hormonal dance can be a revelation—especially if you've been suffering from the effects of imbalanced hormones without realizing it. The more you know about your hormones, the more empowered you are to make healthy choices that nurture and support their equilibrium. If you discover that any are low or imbalanced, it may be a breakthrough on your way to maximizing your hormonal health and enhancing your sexuality.

You can evaluate your hormones with a variety of approaches; the first is simply through your own general observation. The preceding descriptions of the roles your hormones play in your body—their benefits when you have healthy levels, and the symptoms if you don't—can help to give you an overall sense of whether or not you have an imbalance of any of them. If you have symptoms, you can use the following chart to help ascertain which of your hormones may be low. The check marks give you a profile of the typical symptom pattern for deficiencies of each hormone.

113

Do you have the symptoms below?	Low Estrogen	Low Progesterone	Low DHEA	Low Testosterone	Low Cortisol	Low Thyroid
Decreased sexual desire	✓	✓	✓	✓	✓	✓
Decreased sexual response	✓	✓	✓	✓	✓	✓
Difficulty achieving orgasm	✓	✓	✓	✓	✓	✓
Dry and/or thin skin	✓			✓		✓
Head hair that is thinning or falling out	✓					✓
Fatigue	✓	✓	✓	✓	✓	✓
Breast swelling or tenderness		✓				✓
Vaginal and vulvar dryness	✓			✓		✓
Vaginal/vulvar pain with intercourse	✓		✓	✓		✓
Hot flashes or night sweats	✓	✓	✓	✓	✓	✓
Gaining weight easily	✓	✓		✓		✓
Difficulty losing weight	✓		✓	✓		✓
Depression	✓	✓	✓	✓	✓	✓
Anxiety associated with menstrual cycle	✓	✓				
Chronically cold hands and feet						✓

Do you have the symptoms below?	Low Estrogen	Low Progesterone	Low DHEA	Low Testosterone	Low Cortisol	Low Thyroid
Permanent "goose bumps," or dry, bumpy skin on the backs of arms						✓
Insomnia	✓	✓	✓		✓	✓
Chronic allergies			✓		✓	✓
Low blood sugar episodes			✓		✓	✓
Constipation	✓					✓
Water retention or edema						✓
Irregular menstrual cycles	✓	✓				✓
Heavy periods		✓				✓
Very light periods	✓	✓				
Decreased stress tolerance	✓	✓	✓	✓	✓	✓
Urinary incontinence	✓		✓	✓	✓	
General aches and pains	✓	✓	✓	✓		✓
Poor memory	✓	✓	✓	✓	✓	✓
Heart palpitations	✓	✓		✓	✓	✓

Although this chart may help identify whether you have hormone imbalances, some imbalances can be difficult to detect and their symptoms subtle. To more definitively determine if your hormones are imbalanced, you can have a doctor order laboratory tests. These tests aren't recommended for every woman, but if the preceding chart indicates that you have hormone imbalances, you may benefit from them—especially if you experience exaggerated PMS, abnormal menstrual cycles, or menopausal symptoms. There are a number of ways to test your hormones; see Appendix E to learn more about the most comprehensive and accurate methods available.

Enhancing Your Sexuality by Solving Hormone-Related Imbalances

As you've explored, your hormones play enormously influential roles in your body, mind, and spirit, and can affect every facet of how you feel. If your hormones aren't in harmony, *you* won't be either; imbalances can take a huge toll on your sexuality, health, and quality of life, and in some cases transform your hormones from libido-boosters to libido-busters.

If you continually experience adrenal-gland fatigue, for example, you're not apt to feel especially sexy or vital. Your body may lack the extra reserves it needs to nourish vibrant health and sexual vigor. Many women live in a perpetual state of hormonal mayhem, and have no idea what's causing their discomforts. Common hormone-related conditions that can noticeably interfere with your sex life include PMS, heavy menstrual flow, and adrenal and thyroid disorders. Later in the chapter we'll also consider the special class of hormonal swings associated with midlife.

There's a lot you can do to prevent or treat all of these conditions. Many can be resolved with simple lifestyle shifts and nutritional, herbal, or hormonal supplementation. Some women need additional support because of their unique situations, but regardless of what condition you may need to solve, you can improve your hormonal harmony and sexual energy by strengthening your foundation of health with the plan laid out in Chapters 1 and 2.

This is vividly reflected in the view of traditional Chinese medicine. As touched on earlier in this book, when you have abundant chi, you're more likely to enjoy balanced hormones and healthy sexuality. Deficient chi leads to diminished libido, lethargy, depression, heavy periods, infertility, postpartum depression, and symptoms of adrenal-gland fatigue and low thyroid hormone. Chi can be restored through a more restful lifestyle and a healthy balance of yin and yang energy.

In Chapter 3, we looked at another common chi imbalance known as "stuck chi"—an inefficient flow of chi—which can also reduce the quality of your sex life. In addition, it can cause pain, masses such as cysts and fibroids, heavy menstrual flow (especially with clotting), irritability and frustration associated with PMS, and erratic emotions during menopausal changes. If you have stuck chi, exercise can be a highly effective way to get it flowing again.

In the following pages you'll discover many ways you can enhance your sexual health and nourish your libido by solving common hormone imbalances, and resolve deficient or stuck chi, with herbs, flower essences, or acupressure. In addition to solutions for PMS, heavy menstrual flow, adrenal issues, and thyroid imbalances, special attention will be given to menopausal hormone changes, since they're the most likely cause of low libido during many women's lives. The tools and medicines we'll explore are both modern and ancient, but all are *natural* solutions designed to *harmonize*, not harm, your hormones and your health.

Transforming PMS:
From Premenstrual Syndrome to Premenstrual Sex

Many women think of PMS as the classic libido bane, and have no idea that it can often be prevented or successfully treated. They simply resign themselves to the belief that as long as they menstruate, they'll have to spend part of every month dealing with unpleasant physical and emotional symptoms.

If you share this view, it's understandable. Conventional medicine sees PMS largely as unavoidable and unpreventable. This erroneous idea can be especially unfortunate if you're one of the many women who have sought professional help for symptoms of PMS. You may have been prescribed birth-control pills or an antidepressant like Prozac, with unsatisfactory results—and serious side effects.

If you're the typical woman who experiences PMS, your symptoms may last for a week—although for some women PMS can last up to two weeks—and subside when your menstrual flow begins. The symptoms can hamper your sex life for good reason: they may include fatigue, headaches, insomnia, acne, food cravings, weight gain, water retention and bloating, breast swelling and tenderness, mood swings, depression, irritability, impatience, frustration, weepiness, and hypersensitivity. You may feel unable to deal with your normal responsibilities and experience increasing anxiety as you approach the end of your menstrual cycle. The emotional symptoms, which can vary in severity, are notorious for making sex unlikely; you may find your partner's idiosyncrasies not only unattractive but irritating (and he may naturally find you equally exasperating at this time of month).

The libido-limiting potential of PMS makes preventing or treating it all the more important. If you experience PMS for a week each month during your menstruating years, you could spend a combined total of about seven years of your life coping with its symptoms. Solving PMS can open many doors, allowing you to experience the time before you menstruate as positive and pleasurable, rather than condemned to inevitable negativity and pain. You may be surprised to discover that during this part of your cycle you can be not only symptom-free but sexually fulfilled—and find that your partner's idiosyncrasies are really quite lovable after all.

PMS is largely preventable or treatable because *it* isn't the problem; it's a constellation of symptoms that reflects underlying imbalances in your body. These can be due to your stress levels, neurotransmitters, and other factors, but the most frequent causes are hormone imbalances. Numerous studies show that balancing your hormones can be essential to resolving symptoms of PMS. Imbalances in estrogen and progesterone are among the common culprits; as this chapter has pointed out, estrogen dominance—too much estrogen relative to progesterone—can increase PMS symptoms. Cortisol and thyroid-hormone imbalances can also cause the symptoms, as well as hormone imbalances in the years leading up to menopause, when women typically experience drops in hormone levels.

You can use the hormone-evaluation and hormone-testing techniques outlined earlier (and in Appendix E) to determine if hormone imbalances are implicated in your PMS symptoms. If you have estrogen dominance, you can treat PMS by boosting your progesterone level with methods we'll explore in the following pages. With estrogen dominance, your PMS symptoms are likely to include breast swelling and tenderness, bloating, headaches, and heavy menstrual flow. Estrogen dominance can be the result of your liver not breaking down this hormone efficiently, so you can also treat your symptoms by enhancing your estrogen metabolism. Later in this chapter, you'll discover how to accomplish this with dietary choices and supplementation.

Cortisol and thyroid-hormone imbalances can contribute to PMS because they're important in the functioning of all your hormones—especially those pertaining to ovulation and the release of progesterone. If your PMS is due to imbalances of either cortisol or thyroid hormone, you can treat your symptoms by following the recommendations you'll find later in this chapter for addressing adrenal and thyroid imbalances.

You don't have to live with untreated PMS. There's a lot you can do to tackle the underlying causes and prevent its decidedly unsexy symptoms. Let's look at several steps you can take to treat PMS—some that are well-known approaches, and a few that are "secrets." The first two are applicable if low progesterone is contributing to your symptoms; the others can help if your symptoms are due to other causes.

— **Chaste-tree berry.** If you're low in progesterone but would rather not take hormones, chaste-tree berry can be particularly beneficial for treating PMS. This herb is known as a *phyto-progesterone* because of its ability to promote your body's progesterone production. (Despite its name, it won't make you chaste; to the contrary, it can enhance your sex life by helping you treat PMS.) The recommend daily dose is 40 drops of liquid extract, or 175 mg of standardized powdered extract.

— **Natural bioidentical progesterone.** Many women respond well to taking natural bioidentical progesterone for symptoms of PMS due to low progesterone. It should be taken from midcycle (approximately day 14) until your menstrual flow begins (usually around day 28). It's best applied to your skin as a transdermal oil or cream (later in this chapter, you'll find a description of these, and Appendix F contains detailed information on using them). Typical doses of natural bioidentical progesterone for PMS are between 25 and 100 mg taken each night before bed, although a dose as low as 12 mg may be all you need to mitigate your symptoms and enhance your sexuality.

— **Lifestyle therapy.** Following the Great Sex Lifestyle mapped out earlier in this book helps keep your hormones in balance and PMS under control. Make sure you take your daily supplements, especially your multivitamin, and avoid caffeine; research shows that excessive caffeine makes PMS symptoms more likely. Regular exercise can reduce symptoms by lowering your estrogen level, increasing your circulation, elevating your endorphin production, and helping you fight depression. Minimize your stress level; if stress is unavoidable, manage it wisely. The Great Sex Detox in Chapter 2 further promotes your body's ability to keep PMS at bay.

— **Extra supplement support.** Whatever multivitamin or other supplements you take, make sure you get 50 mg of vitamin B_6, 1,000 mg of calcium, and 500 mg of magnesium daily. If one of your PMS symptoms is depression, take 1,000 mg of the amino acid tyrosine daily. (Tyrosine should be taken in the morning.)

— **Saint-John's-wort.** If you have PMS symptoms of weepiness, depression, and major mood shifts, an underlying cause may be a low level of your "feel-good" neurotransmitter serotonin. As you discovered previously in this chapter, your estrogen and serotonin levels rise and fall together. When your estrogen level subsides toward the end of your cycle, your serotonin level also drops, making you much more prone to mood swings and depression before your periods. The herb Saint-John's-wort can help alleviate these PMS symptoms—ample research has shown its effectiveness in treating depression—which in turn can allow you greater opportunities to experience pleasure. The recommended daily dose is 900 mg standardized to contain 0.3 percent hypericin. (Note: Saint-John's-wort may affect the actions of certain prescription medications.)

—**Xiao Yao Wan.** In Chinese medicine, symptoms of PMS are often accompanied by a diagnosis of "liver chi stagnation," which means your chi isn't circulating freely through your liver and throughout your body. If you have this condition, your PMS symptoms typically include a high level of irritability, frustration, and anger, as well as swollen, painful breasts. The Chinese herbal formula known as Xiao Yao Wan, or Free and Easy Wanderer, which was mentioned in the preceding chapter as a treatment for menstrual cramps, can effectively move your chi and boost your libido at the same time. It can reduce irritability and anger before your periods, and help you feel relaxed, content, and as its name suggests, free and easy. It's made by many companies, and dosages vary; follow the recommendations on the product label. (See Appendix C for supplier information.)

— **Aromatherapy.** The essential oil bergamot, a lovely musky-smelling citrus oil, can help you relax, balance your emotions, and gently relieve PMS symptoms. Bergamot is recommended if you've been under excessive stress or have trouble expressing your emotions, and it's also used to stimulate libido blocked by depression and frustration. You can apply it with a spray dispenser to your chest and abdomen twice a day to help allay symptoms. (Bergamot can increase your skin's photosensitivity, so refrain from using it before you're exposed to sunlight.)

— **Acupressure.** As you've discovered, "stuck chi" can lead to pain and emotional irritability, and lower the quality of your sex life. The acupressure point Liver 3 can be especially helpful for PMS because it gets your chi moving again; it's also known in Chinese medicine as *Great Thoroughfare*, due to its importance as a conduit for the flow of chi. To relieve symptoms of PMS and support your sexual energy as well, you or your partner can press firmly on this point for one to three minutes, at least twice daily as needed. For added impact, bergamot can be applied to the point; this may stimulate the point and help keep your chi moving. (To locate the Liver 3 point, see Appendix A.)

— **Flower essences.** By helping create subtle emotional shifts and engender calm, peaceful feelings, flower essences can be a soothing way of supporting other approaches to preventing and relieving PMS. The flower essence known as *impatiens* can help you stabilize your emotions if you're feeling impatient, agitated, burned-out, hurried, and harried. It nurtures your ability to slow down, relax, be centered in the moment, and get in touch with your feelings—including feelings of sensuality. Another flower essence, *cayenne,* can help you move past feelings of being emotionally blocked, and gain a sense of new, forward-moving growth and energy in your life. Flower essences can be taken every few hours until symptoms subside (usually within 12 hours); the typical dose is a few pellets or drops under your tongue.

Unburdening Your Libido from Heavy Menstrual Flow

If you have heavy "moon flow," it can drain your energy and libido, even if it's not accompanied by painful cramping. Alleviating heavy menstrual flow can make a big difference in how you experience your periods, and create new possibilities for your sexual energy (which doesn't necessarily have to involve sex). A segment of your cycle you once thought doomed to the discomforts of "bad moons" can instead become a positive time in your life.

Heavy menstrual bleeding has the potential to dramatically decrease your libido because it can lead to anemia due to iron deficiency. Iron, a mineral incorporated into your red blood cells, allows oxygen to be carried to every cell in your body. You need iron and oxygen not only to sustain your life and perform your body's functions, but also to convert the amino acid tyrosine into dopamine, a brain chemical that enables you to feel pleasure. If you're chronically anemic because of heavy menstrual bleeding, inadequate dopamine can make you susceptible to lower libido and diminished sexual response, along with feelings of worthlessness and hopelessness.

As you explored earlier in this chapter, ancient practitioners of Chinese medicine referred to a woman's menstrual flow as her Heavenly Water. From a traditional Chinese medical perspective, if you have heavy Heavenly Water, it's due to a chi deficiency, and if you have blood clotting as well, it's the result of stuck chi. From a modern Western perspective, the underlying causes of heavy menstrual bleeding and clotting are often hormone imbalances. By addressing the underlying causes of the condition, from both an Eastern and Western standpoint, you can lift the heaviness from your Heavenly Water and transform your periods.

The most common hormone imbalances that can cause heavy menstrual bleeding involve your estrogen and progesterone levels. As you've discovered, progesterone plays a key role in preventing the estrogen in your body from being too prolific, and helps keep the endometrial lining that builds up in your uterus every month from becoming too thick. Since the endometrial lining sloughs off and becomes your menstrual flow, having adequate progesterone can keep your Heavenly Water light.

Heavy menstrual flow can be due to another common hormone imbalance—a low thyroid-hormone level. As you've seen, you can have low thyroid hormone even if laboratory blood testing says you're normal—a condition known as "subclinically low" thyroid hormone. (See Appendix E for more information on thyroid-hormone testing.) If you have heavy menstrual flow and low thyroid hormone, you may benefit from nutritional support for your thyroid gland and natural thyroid-hormone medication. Some women with low thyroid hormone, including some who are subclinically low, have less menstrual bleeding—as well as more regular cycles, improved ability to lose weight, and increased libido—when taking nutritional supplements and natural thyroid-hormone medication.

Hormone imbalances can lead to other conditions that can cause you to have heavy menstrual flow, including uterine polyps, uterine fibroids, and ovarian cysts. If you have heavy menstrual flow, it's recommended that you see a gynecologist for a thorough evaluation to rule out these and other conditions.

Let's look at ways you can help restore your sexual response throughout your cycle by lightening your Heavenly Water:

— **Natural bioidentical progesterone.** If you have heavy bleeding due to low progesterone, you may stand to gain from taking natural bioidentical progesterone, applied to your skin as a transdermal oil or cream. The recommended dose is between 25 and 100 mg, taken each night at bedtime during the second half of your cycle. (You'll find guidelines for applying transdermal progesterone later in this chapter and in Appendix F.)

— **Thyroid support.** As mentioned above, in the event that you have heavy bleeding along with low thyroid hormone—and this applies whether you're subclinically low or not—you can gain from taking nutritional support for your thyroid gland, as well as from natural thyroid medication. Nutritional support consists of supplementation with tyrosine, iodine, and selenium; and natural thyroid medication may include a product such as Armour Thyroid or Naturthroid. Descriptions of all of these appear in the following pages in our discussion of thyroid imbalances; the dose amounts and other recommendations suggested there are appropriate for treating heavy menstrual flow associated with low thyroid hormone.

— **Tips from Chinese medicine.** According to Chinese medicine, you can treat heavy menstrual flow by correcting the chi deficiency that causes it. You can strengthen your chi through the Great Sex Lifestyle recommended earlier in this book and by balancing your hormones. Healthy lifestyle choices also keep the chi circulating in your pelvis, which can make a big difference in the quality of your menstrual flow by alleviating the stuck chi that causes clotting. You can also treat heavy menstrual bleeding by taking Chinese herbal formulas before your Heavenly Water begins flowing each month. To have a formula made specifically for you, see a qualified practitioner of Chinese herbal medicine. (See Appendix B.) One standard formula, known as Myomin, available from Chinese herbalists and online, combines four herbs to treat heavy bleeding due to excess estrogen by lowering your estrogen level. The recommended dose is two pills twice daily.

Acupressure can also treat heavy menstrual flow by strengthening your chi; press on your Spleen 6 point for one to three minutes each day. To move your chi and treat clotting with heavy menstrual bleeding, press on your Liver 3 point for one to three minutes each day. (See Appendix A to locate both points.)

If you have heavy menstrual flow that leads to anemia due to iron deficiency, two other useful options should be mentioned here. While these don't directly address the causes of heavy menstrual bleeding, they can play a supportive role by helping you overcome related issues that can get in the way of your sexuality.

— **Ba Zhen Wan.** Chinese medicine holds that chronic anemia leads to a chi deficiency, and many herbal formulas can help you recover from anemia and restore your chi. One of the best, called Ba Zhen Wan, or "Women's Precious Pills," is available through Chinese herbalists and online. (For supplier information, see Appendix C.) The formula is made by many companies; take the recommended dose on the product label, and continue taking it for at least six months to rebuild your chi.

To reinforce the effects of Women's Precious Pills, you can do acupressure for anemia and chi deficiency. Press the following points for one to three minutes each day: Ren 6, Ren 12, Spleen 6, Liver 8, Stomach 36, and Large Intestine 11. (To locate these points, see Appendix A.)

— **Additional supplement support.** If your heavy menstrual flow results in anemia due to iron deficiency, in addition to taking 40 mg of iron daily, you may benefit from taking the amino acid tyrosine. Although tyrosine doesn't address anemia itself, as a precursor to dopamine it assists with your dopamine level and supports your ability to experience pleasure. (Note: To properly convert tyrosine into dopamine, you need to have adequate iron and oxygen in your body.) The recommended daily dose is 1,000 mg taken in the morning. Some women feel revved up when they begin taking tyrosine, so it's best to start with a low dose and increase it gradually. If you're already taking tyrosine as outlined above for symptoms of depression with PMS or for heavy menstrual bleeding associated with low thyroid hormone, you won't need to take more.

Addressing Adrenal Challenges: The Sexual Benefits

Your adrenal glands are essential for your health and libido; they give you energy you need for everything in your life, including sex. In addition, they improve your tolerance for stress, especially during challenging phases of your life, and help sustain you through the hormonal transitions of midlife.

If your sex life is waning as a result of long-term unrelenting stress, you may suffer from *adrenal fatigue*—a condition in which your adrenal glands become exhausted and unable to function properly. This is often due to a prolonged experience of excessive work without sufficient time to rest and recuperate, and not enough time spent simply enjoying life. If you have this condition, you may feel completely "spent," devoid of sexual energy, and as if you simply have nothing left to give. Because adrenal fatigue can have so many undesirable effects on desire, solving it can vastly improve your potential for pleasure.

As we've elaborated on in this chapter, your adrenal glands produce cortisol, a key player in your hormonal dance and a vital factor for your libido. One of the most important aspects of maintaining your sexual energy is supporting your adrenal glands in their day-to-day cortisol production. Steady, balanced cortisol provides many benefits for your health and allows you to fully enjoy your sexuality, but too much or too little can drain your libido and leave you feeling burned-out. Chronically high cortisol production can eventually cause your adrenal glands to become fatigued because they simply can't sustain that level of stress-hormone output; this can ultimately lead to adrenal-gland exhaustion and, paradoxically, *low* cortisol production, resulting in chronic fatigue and lack of energy. This is why continuously elevated cortisol production is linked with many other health issues, including suppressed immunity, irregular menstrual cycles, weight gain, anxiety, and low sexual response.

If you have adrenal fatigue, you may need adrenal support to balance your cortisol, restore your energy, and stimulate your libido. It can be especially beneficial if your life is demanding, you're under a high level of stress, and you need that extra "push," day after day. You can support your adrenal health on a short-term basis—it can help you weather the storm of finals week, or a period of stressful travel—but in order to increase your sex drive, adrenal support should be undertaken long-term. By nurturing your adrenal health over time, you can gradually replenish your depleted sexual energy.

You can begin supporting your adrenal glands by making the right lifestyle choices. First and foremost, manage stress wisely. Some is unavoidable, but you can choose how you respond to it and whether to take on new stressful projects in your life. Create a lifestyle that gives you plenty of time to relax and rejuvenate. Remember to stop and smell the roses, and incorporate gentle, yin exercises into your daily routines. You can accomplish your goals, but not without adequate downtime. Pushing yourself every day eventually becomes counterproductive by triggering the high cortisol production that can result in adrenal fatigue, chronic exhaustion, low sexual energy, insomnia, and other symptoms.

Your dietary choices can also bolster your sex drive by supporting your adrenal function. Make sure you eat three meals and at least two snacks a day to keep your blood sugar even; if you skip meals, your cortisol may rise to an unhealthy level to compensate for a lack of sugar to "feed" your brain. As you discovered in Chapter 2, it's best to eat foods with a low glycemic index. High-glycemic foods like sugary doughnuts cause your body to release excessive insulin, resulting in a subsequent drop in blood sugar that leaves you feeling hungry, tired, and craving more sugar. Your body then releases more cortisol, in a vicious cycle that keeps you in a perpetual state of adrenal fatigue.

You can further enhance your adrenal function by avoiding foods that cause allergic reactions. When you consume a food allergen, the effects can be similar to those of eating high-glycemic sugary foods: an insulin surge results in low blood sugar, then a spike in your cortisol level, and you may wind up feeling fatigued, shaky, and craving sweets.

Herbs, supplements, and natural bioidentical hormones can also help to buoy your adrenal glands and support your libido. Let's look at the most effective options, beginning with two adrenal-supportive herbs. In the next chapter, you'll discover more herbal remedies (including Chinese "sexual tonics") that have the ability to further boost your adrenal function.

— **Siberian ginseng.** For centuries, this herb has been used to strengthen the body, boost health, and increase longevity. Modern science has confirmed its benefits: Siberian ginseng contains compounds that can help you overcome stress by supporting your adrenal glands' hormone production, as well as stimulate your immune system to help fight off infections. (One study found it effective in reducing herpes outbreaks.) Siberian ginseng may also increase your mental alertness, energy, sense of well-being, and sex drive.

For supporting your adrenal glands to enhance your libido, the recommended dose is 100 to 200 mg, containing a standardized extract of 0.5 percent eleutheroside, taken two to three times daily. Siberian ginseng has very few unfavorable side effects and is safe for lactating women. Some people experience slight diarrhea if they take an excessive amount or insomnia if they take it near bedtime. Those who have uncontrolled high blood pressure or are taking barbiturates or the drug digoxin shouldn't use it.

— *Rhodiola rosea.* This potent herb has long been used in folk medicine to foster fertility, physical endurance, energy, and longevity, and to alleviate maladies of the nervous system. A large body of scientific research has validated its health-enhancing effects; for example, it can improve your capacity for mental and physical exertion, and reduce your recovery time after intense exercise. Rhodiola is known as an *adaptogen* because it assists you in adapting to stress—which is why it's so beneficial in fighting adrenal fatigue and diminished libido. It helps you beat stress by affecting levels of hormones and neurotransmitters your body releases in response to stressful situations. It can also inhibit the breakdown of neurotransmitters such as dopamine, serotonin, and norepinephrine—all of which can enhance your sex drive.

Studies suggest that rhodiola can have other beneficial effects on your hormonal system as well—for instance, by supporting your thyroid-gland function (which in turn further protects your adrenal glands from being overburdened), and enhancing your immunity through its actions on your thymus gland. Research also indicates that rhodiola may boost fertility by improving egg maturation and increasing the number of follicles (vesicles that contain developing eggs) growing in the ovaries.

Many people who take rhodiola find that it elevates their energy, moods, mental clarity, and sexuality. For adrenal and libido support, the recommended daily dose is 100 to 170 mg in a standardized form containing 2.6 percent rosavin. Rhodiola is considered a very safe herb, but its rare side effects include insomnia and anxiety. It shouldn't be used by anyone taking antidepressants or stimulants, or those with bipolar disorders.

— **Vitamin C.** When you go through acute or chronic stress, you can lose a lot of vitamin C through your urine; if you experience stress-induced adrenal fatigue, be sure you're getting an adequate amount of this vital supplement. In addition, vitamin C is important in your body's production of adrenal hormones. If you're under stress and have low adrenal function, take a minimum of 1,000 mg of vitamin C twice daily to support your adrenal health.

— **Pantothenic acid.** Also known as vitamin B_5, pantothenic acid plays a key role in your body's production of adrenal hormones. If you have adrenal fatigue due to stress, the recommended dose is 250 mg twice daily.

— **Phosphatidylserine.** This supplement derived from soy can improve your body's ability to handle the symptoms of anxiety or insomnia often linked with excessive stress, a high cortisol level, and adrenal fatigue. If your cortisol level is too high during the day, you may be subject to anxiety; if it's too high at night, you may be prone to insomnia. You can reduce anxiety associated with stress-induced high cortisol by taking phosphatidylserine during the day. To prevent insomnia associated with stress-induced high cortisol, take it before bedtime. The recommended dose is 90 to 180 mg daily. Phosphatidylserine is well tolerated by most people, and should be taken along with a high-protein snack.

— **Progesterone.** If you experience the libido-restricting effects of adrenal fatigue due to stress, you may benefit appreciably from taking natural bioidentical progesterone. As you saw in the "hormone cascade" diagram, progesterone acts as a precursor to cortisol. Because of this, it supports your adrenal glands in their daily cortisol production, enhancing your health and sexual energy.

Taking natural bioidentical progesterone can also increase progesterone's other benefits in your body. For example, it can help in midlife when your ovaries significantly reduce their hormone production and start looking for a new "career." At this point, as we've touched on previously, your adrenal glands suddenly find themselves promoted to the job of taking over where your ovaries left off—one more reason why you'll gain from having strong adrenal health.

The amount of progesterone you need, and how long you should take it, depends on your individual requirements and situation. Natural progesterone creams are found at health-food stores, but for best results, see a licensed naturopathic doctor or other qualified holistic practitioner for guidance; taking natural progesterone without first getting an assessment of your entire hormonal system can create more imbalance. It's most effective when used as a transdermal (applied to your skin) oil or cream each night before you go to bed. You should take natural progesterone only if you need it and begin with a low dose, then slowly build up to the dose that works best for you. Recommended daily doses for adrenal and libido support typically range from 25 to 100 mg. (Later in this chapter, you'll find guidelines for using transdermal progesterone, and additional information in Appendix F.)

— **DHEA.** You can also use natural bioidentical DHEA to address the effects of stress-induced adrenal fatigue and low sexual energy. The "hormone cascade" diagram earlier in this chapter shows how DHEA, like progesterone, is a precursor to cortisol, which means that it, too, supports your adrenal glands in producing cortisol and enhancing your health and libido. In addition, taking natural DHEA can promote the other benefits of DHEA that we explored earlier—whether you're in midlife, or at any other time. To take DHEA for adrenal support, apply 4 to 8 mg daily to your skin (preferably to your labia) as a transdermal oil or cream. Start with a low dose and increase the amount only if needed; too much DHEA in your body can have undesirable effects. You can purchase DHEA at health-food stores, but for best results, seek the guidance of a licensed naturopathic doctor or other appropriate practitioner.

Liberating Your Libido from Thyroid Imbalances

As you've discovered, your thyroid gland is a powerhouse for your libido; your thyroid hormone helps generate the energy you need for everything you do, sexually and otherwise. But although the benefits of a balanced thyroid-hormone level are multifaceted, if you have too much or too little, it can throw off your capacity for sexual pleasure and pervade your health with a wide range of adverse repercussions.

Identifying and correcting low thyroid hormone can be crucial not only to your sexuality and overall quality of life, but also for keeping the rest of your hormonal system in balance and working well. If you experience many of the symptoms that show check marks for low thyroid hormone on the "hormone symptom chart" that appeared earlier in this chapter, it's a good idea to begin your own therapy by supporting your thyroid health with nutritional supplements. You can take the following supplements to help rectify a low thyroid level and revitalize your sex life:

— **Tyrosine.** This amino acid gives your thyroid gland the nutrition it needs to manufacture your thyroid hormones T4 and T3. The recommended daily dose is 1,000 mg taken in the morning. Tyrosine can have a stimulating effect when you first begin taking it, so you should start with a lower amount and gradually work up to this dose.

— **Iodine.** A mineral critical to your body's ability to produce thyroid hormones, iodine is plentiful in many seafoods, seaweeds, and iodized salt. (If you don't have sufficient iodine, you're prone to developing a benign thyroid tumor known as a goiter.) As a supplement, the recommended daily dose is 150 mcg for females age 11 or older, 175 mcg for pregnant women, and 200 mcg for breast-feeding mothers. (Note: People with Hashimoto's thyroiditis or Graves' disease should refrain from taking iodine.)

— **Selenium.** An important mineral for your thyroid health, selenium supports the conversion of the inactive thyroid hormone (T4) into the active thyroid hormone (T3). The recommended daily dose is 200 mcg.

❖ ❖ ❖

Supporting your thyroid health with these supplements may be enough to remedy a low thyroid-hormone level (they can all be taken at the same time), and you may not need additional treatment. But if your symptoms persist, you should find professional guidance to further gauge your thyroid-hormone status. You can gather useful information by having a physician order the tests described earlier in this chapter and delineated in Appendix E—although, as we mentioned, you may have low thyroid hormone even if testing indicates you're normal. If test results are normal but your symptoms continue, see a naturopathic physician for a more complete assessment and to help ascertain if you have subclinically low thyroid hormone. Either way—whether your low thyroid level is revealed by testing, or you're subclinically low—taking thyroid-hormone medication can give your body the ideal thyroid support it may need. Let's look at the keys to using thyroid-hormone medication to elevate your thyroid level and your libido:

— **Thyroid-hormone medication . . . what you need to know.** If a doctor diagnoses you as having low thyroid hormone (hypothyroidism), there's a good chance that you'll benefit from taking thyroid hormones. They're available by prescription only, but conventionally trained medical doctors are unlikely to tell you about all of your options.

There are two types of thyroid-hormone replacement: natural and synthetic. Patients diagnosed by medical doctors as being low-thyroid are typically prescribed only synthetic thyroid hormone, such as Synthroid or Levothyroxine. Some people respond well to these products, but others continue to experience fatigue and other symptoms of low thyroid hormone.

In addition to the philosophical issue—you probably prefer a natural to a synthetic treatment—there's a real practical difference between natural and synthetic thyroid-hormone medication. The natural option contains both the inactive form of thyroid hormone (T4) and the active form (T3), but the synthetic option contains only T4. So if you take natural instead of synthetic thyroid hormone, it can make a huge difference in how you feel and the results you get. As previously mentioned, T3 stimulates your cells to produce energy, so the natural option may more effectively help restore your energy level and libido, especially if you don't convert your T4 to T3 very well.

A licensed naturopathic physician or other qualified holistically oriented practitioner can thoroughly evaluate your thyroid-hormone needs and help you determine if you should be on natural thyroid-hormone medication. If you've been prescribed synthetic thyroid medication by a conventional practitioner, but you still often feel tired or experience other symptoms of low thyroid hormone that we outlined earlier in this chapter, you may benefit from natural thyroid-hormone medication such as Armour Thyroid or Naturthroid. It could be just what you've been waiting for to revitalize your energy level and sex drive.

The amount of natural thyroid medication you take, and how long you take it, will be determined by your doctor to suit your unique needs. With any type of thyroid-hormone medication, the lowest dose needed is generally best. Armour Thyroid and Naturthroid are typically taken daily in pill form, about 20 minutes before breakfast.

If your thyroid-hormone level is too high, you should be guided in your treatment options by a licensed naturopathic doctor or other holistic practitioner. High-thyroid conditions, which include Hashimoto's thyroiditis and Graves' disease, can be complex and are beyond the scope of this book.

Hormones and Infertility: The Sex Connection

If you've been diagnosed with infertility, you may be surprised to discover that many of the steps you can take to address infertility also enhance your sexuality. For conception to happen, you need the healthy, harmonious hormones that promote a strong libido. If you have any of the hormone-related imbalances we've explored in this chapter—including estrogen dominance (which may be associated with abnormal or absent ovulation), adrenal fatigue, or a low thyroid-hormone level—solving them can be crucial to successful conception. For example, if your progesterone or DHEA levels are low, taking natural progesterone or DHEA may help you conceive.

About 20 percent of couples unable to conceive are diagnosed with "unexplained infertility." In some of these cases, it may be because the woman has a subclinically low thyroid-hormone level (low thyroid hormone that doesn't show up on tests), and she may conceive when her thyroid imbalance has been addressed.

All of the lifestyle factors you explored earlier in this book for enhancing your sexuality also help to address infertility by supporting balanced hormones. Your Great Sex Detox, as spelled out in Chapter 2,
could be particularly relevant here. The hormone-mimicking chemicals
ubiquitous in the environment, also known as *hormone-disrupters,* may
play an especially important role for many would-be parents. (They affect some couples more than others because each person can react
differently to them—depending in part on genetic makeup—but decreasing exposure to these chemicals can help create hormonal balance
and enhance fertility.)

Intrauterine insemination and in vitro fertilization can help increase
the likelihood of conception, but any couple seeking help for unexplained infertility should first restore great health and vitality in their
bodies. This echoes ancient Chinese medicine, which teaches that infertility can be caused by chi imbalances; a lifestyle that supports chi,
and allows sexual chi to flourish, is essential for conception to happen.
No amount of hormonal manipulation with fertility drugs can correct
underlying chi imbalances.

Mastering Menopause: Sex in Your Second Spring

The transition you experience in midlife marks the beginning
of a period of great potential creativity and rebirth. Your changing
hormones not only affect you physically, but also influence your
thoughts and feelings, so your menopausal metamorphosis can be
a time of renewal for your body, mind, and spirit—and a time of
sexual discovery.

You don't have to accept the negative connotations that the
word *menopause* may have for some people—as if it's only a time of
uncontrollable hormone shifts, difficult symptoms, and loss of libido. You can embrace midlife as an opportunity to fulfill new expectations about your body, your sexuality, and your well-being.
One postmenopausal patient described her midlife experience as
"giving birth to my older, wiser self, and being set free from the
old me . . . along with some of the most gratifying sexual experiences of my lifetime, and sensations of sexual 'newness' and well-
being that I haven't felt since my teenage years."

The notion that menopause is a time of regeneration and
spiritual rebirth may seem unfathomable to some practitioners of
conventional Western medicine, but it has been widely held for
thousands of years in Chinese medicine. In fact, in the traditional

Chinese view, your midlife transition is known as your "Second Spring." According to this outlook, every month between puberty and menopause your chi flows downward toward the earth, from your heart to your uterus, to produce menstrual blood (your Heavenly Water) and give you the potential to bear and nourish children. If this downward flow of chi and blood continued past midlife, your chi would become depleted and you would age prematurely. Instead, at midlife your body conserves your chi by reversing the flow; it begins flowing upward, from your uterus to your heart, away from the earth and toward your spirit. No longer devoted to the possibility of bearing and nourishing children, your chi can be used to bear and nourish your spirit. Menopause is seen as a time of liberated energy and joy, when your upward-flowing chi lifts your spirit to new heights, giving you vast opportunities for self-development and expanding your spiritual potential. One Chinese medical authority describes it as the time when you become a wellspring of wisdom and a mother figure in your community. Your Second Spring is the passage of your energy from Heavenly Water to heavenly wisdom.

By challenging the conventional Western view of menopause, you can not only experience it as a time of heightened consciousness and spiritual awakening, but you can also open up an entire phase of your life—which some medical "experts" may have written off as destined for discomfort and diminished libido—to new possibilities for sexual pleasure instead. And like many women, you may find that menopause brings a newfound sense of sexual freedom, not only because you no longer have to be concerned about birth control, but because without the hormonal ups and downs of menstrual cycles, you may have more sustained, steady sexual energy.

Menopause can also provide you with opportunities for profound psychological and spiritual growth because it's the other end of the menstrual spectrum that began in adolescence with your first period. Like adolescence, menopause is a dramatic hormonal transition that enables you to become more aware of your inner rhythms—another window of time that opens up to allow your consciousness to expand.

You may have been living on "autopilot" for much of your adult life, not fully aware of what you really want, or who you actually are. Perhaps your nervous system has been operating within a framework laid down decades ago during your formative years—a framework you once needed to deal with family and social dynamics, but which no longer serves you well. Your menopausal transition gives you the chance to examine this framework and make conscious changes in order to live more in accord with your authentic self—vital for a healthy sex life because it boosts your self-esteem and allows you to claim your own natural sexual needs and make better choices. You can expedite your personal midlife renaissance by keeping a journal, reading self-empowering books, or working with a therapist.

It's important to realize that your experience of menopause is unique; the physical and spiritual changes you go through leading up to and through midlife may be accompanied by a variety of symptoms—or by none at all. If you experience symptoms, they tend to begin in your mid-40s, well before you reach menopause, although some women experience them earlier or later. Menopausal symptoms stem from hormonal imbalances, and not all women are created equally when it comes to midlife hormonal harmony. Some have a tumultuous transition, filled with physical challenges that require much time and attention, while others seem to sail through midlife effortlessly, with little or no difficulty, hardly needing to *pause* for menopause.

If you experience sexual challenges at menopause, it may be due to decreases in your levels of the hormones that nourish the tissues of your pelvis and sex organs; some tissues once well hydrated by your hormones may become drier, and your connective tissues and musculature may become softer. Menopausal symptoms can also compromise your sexuality because, in addition to well-known symptoms such as hot flashes, night sweats, and insomnia, they may resemble exaggerated PMS symptoms—fatigue; headaches; breast tenderness; bloating; mood swings; irritability; depression; and heightened feelings of sensitivity, weepiness, and insecurity. Your periods are apt to become less frequent as you approach menopause, and they may become either much lighter or much heavier. If your hormones fluctuate erratically, you may sometimes feel as if your emotions are riding a crazy roller coaster, and your exaggerated mood swings may be disruptive to your personal relationships, sex life, or career.

The hormone shifts that women experience at midlife can also cause another common symptom—reduced libido. It's not unusual for a menopausal woman to experience little or no interest in sex or intimacy, even though she still loves her partner, and for some couples this can be a source of conflict in their sexual relationship.

If menopausal symptoms pose challenges to your sexuality and health, overcoming them can transform your sex life. There's a tremendous amount that you can do, without synthetic hormones or pharmaceutical drugs, to effectively treat your symptoms, correct hormone imbalances, keep your sex organs healthy, and strengthen your capacity for midlife passion. Let's explore your many options for making your journey through menopause smooth and pleasurable:

Herbs, Nutrition, and Foods to Mitigate Midlife Symptoms and Support Libido

If you're seeking relief from menopausal symptoms, including low libido, you want to begin with the gentlest, weakest, and most conservative measures you can, and gradually move to stronger treatments only if needed. Like some women, you may have low libido but sufficient or borderline hormone levels. These gentle approaches may effectively reduce or eliminate your symptoms, and you may never need any other treatment.

Conventional doctors often jump to the conclusion that if you have menopausal symptoms and a lowered sex drive, you need hormone replacement therapy, largely because their training doesn't adequately prepare them to explore your other options. Hormone replacement therapy has far more potential side effects than other approaches, and it's preferable for your overall health and sexuality if you can avoid them. The following are your best "first line of defense" options for treating menopausal symptoms naturally and gently:

— **Black cohosh.** The herb black cohosh has long been used to alleviate symptoms associated with menopause, including hot flashes, night sweats, depression, and (as you saw earlier in this book) vaginal atrophy and dryness. Research shows that black co-hosh is safe and can be taken for an extended period of time, or until it's no longer necessary for controlling midlife symp-toms. It reduces hot flashes by affecting your estrogen receptors, but doesn't actually increase your estrogen level; this makes it a good choice if you have a family history, or personal history, of estrogen-related cancer. A study published in the journal *Gyne-cological Endocrinology* in 2011 found that black cohosh can also help menopausal women who take the drug tamoxifen (often pre-scribed after breast-cancer diagnoses to prevent future recurrenc-es). Tamoxifen can aggravate menopausal symptoms, but women who took black cohosh in addition had fewer hot flashes, less anx-iety, and improved sleep. The recommended dose of black cohosh for reducing symptoms of menopause is 80 mg taken twice daily.

— **Maca.** A powerful Peruvian herb, maca contains plant sterols that have the ability to strengthen your entire hormonal system. Maca is effective in treating menopausal symptoms of hot flashes, night sweats, and insomnia because it can stimulate your glands to increase their production of estrogen and other hormones—which makes it a valuable alternative to hormone re-placement therapy. Maca has other benefits as well: it supports your adrenal glands, helps lower your stress-hormone level, and increases your sex drive. (It also increases male libido, as you'll dis-cover later in this book.) The recommended dose for menopausal symptoms is 1,000 mg twice daily.

— **Da Bu Yin.** Da Bu Yin is one of the best Chinese herbal for-mulas for treating menopausal symptoms related to a deficiency of yin, which typically include night sweats, insomnia, hot flashes, anxiety, and increased thirst. The herbs in Da Bu Yin have been used for thousands of years and have no known side effects. The recommended dose of one Da Bu Yin product, called Great Yin (see Appendix C), is two to three pills three times daily.

— **Two Immortals.** Also known as *Er Xian Tang,* Two Immor-tals is another traditional Chinese herbal formula for treating menopausal symptoms. It helps to boost libido, balance hormones, relieve hot flashes, and reduce irregular menstrual bleeding and cramping during the years leading up to menopause. It's made by many companies; dosages vary, so follow the recommendation on the product label. (See Appendix C for supplier information.)

— **Vitamin E.** You can help reduce hot flashes by taking vitamin E; the recommended dose is 400 to 800 IU daily. (Take with caution if you're on blood-thinning medication.)

— **Soy.** As a food high in plant hormones, or phytoestrogens, soy can have certain hormone-like effects on your body. Ample research shows that women who consume higher amounts of soy foods experience milder midlife symptoms.

Balancing Your Hormones and Sexuality with Hormone Replacement Therapy

If you've exhausted the possibilities for treatment with herbs, nutritional support, and foods, and still experience menopausal symptoms that compromise your health and sexuality, you may benefit from hormone replacement therapy. Supplementing your body with the right hormones can help restore your hormonal balance, libido, and sexual enthusiasm, and keep your vulva and vagina hydrated. It can also support your immune system, bones, and connective tissues, and by improving your moods, increase your sense of well-being and receptiveness to pleasure.

Whenever possible, you want to use natural bioidentical hormones rather than conventional synthetic hormones, and use the smallest amounts necessary to achieve the desired effects. Natural bioidentical hormones are considered safer than conventional synthetic hormones because they're derived from plant sources and have a chemical structure that's the same as the hormones your body produces over the course of your lifetime (hence the term *bioidentical*). Synthetic hormones can lead to health problems because they rely on forms of hormones structurally very different from those your body naturally makes.

Natural bioidentical hormones are becoming more widely available to help women with menopausal symptoms and low libido—thanks in large part to the alarming results of the 2002 Women's Health Initiative, a long-term study sponsored by the National Institutes of Health that focused on strategies for preventing heart disease, breast cancer, osteoporosis, and colorectal cancer in postmenopausal women. The study showed that conventional hormone replacement therapy can increase your risk for heart disease, stroke, and breast cancer. When these findings were released, many women chose to throw out their conventional hormone prescriptions and suffer the consequences of abrupt mood changes, reduced sex drive, hot flashes, night sweats, insomnia, and other symptoms.

Since then, increasing numbers of women have turned to herbal remedies to ease their symptoms, or sought out natural bioidentical hormone replacement therapy. Research on natural bioidentical hormones has surged, and the growing consensus among experts is that they may be safer for many women. According to a 2009 article in the journal *Postgraduate Medicine*, "data and clinical outcomes demonstrate that bioidentical hormones are associated with lower risks, including the risk of breast cancer and cardiovascular disease, and are more efficacious than their synthetic and animal-derived counterparts." But even though natural bioidentical hormones have become holistically minded doctors' preferred method of hormone replacement therapy, conventional physicians may still encourage you to use synthetic hormones for menopausal symptoms, and especially for decreased libido.

The Women's Health Initiative found that it was women who took Provera and Premarin—at the time the most popular conventional progesterone and estrogen prescriptions for menopausal symptoms—who were at increased risk for dire health consequences. Provera is synthetic and not bioidentical. Premarin, the most well-studied hormone used in conventional hormone replacement therapy, is considered by some to be seminatural—a questionable claim, because it contains 4 to 8 percent horse hormones—and it's certainly not bioidentical. (It may be natural and bioidentical for a horse, but not for *you*. Even though Premarin is derived from another mammal, it contains more than 200 different compounds foreign to your cells. Plant-derived hormones, by contrast, contain natural hormone-like substances that are chemically altered in a laboratory to yield compounds identical to the hormones a woman produces in her body.)

Perhaps it was inevitable that trying to trick Mother Nature with synthetic forms of such powerful substances as hormones would eventually backfire. Many women have similarly put their health on the line by taking synthetic hormones in another form—as birth-control pills. Some take them for their entire reproductive lives, even though it has never been clearly established if their long-term use is safe. Birth-control pills, which contain estrogen and progesterone, interfere with a woman's natural hormone production, suppress ovulation, and can have many other undesirable effects. Some women experience strokes or high blood pressure while taking them, and others develop liver tumors. They may also change the viscosity of your bile, which can lead to the formation of gallstones or have other adverse affects on your gallbladder, resulting in sporadic episodes of painful nausea and vomiting. (For information on natural birth-control methods, see Appendix H.)

The hidden risks of synthetic hormones make natural alternatives all the more attractive. Your options for using natural bioidentical hormones to treat menopausal symptoms and enhance your sexuality have improved considerably since 2002. Today you have many effective choices at your fingertips for taking natural bioidentical estrogen, progesterone, DHEA, and testosterone. You may benefit from using one of them separately, or a combination of several of them. Let's explore your options for therapy with each one:

— **Natural bioidentical estrogen.** The two primary estrogens in your body, as outlined in Appendix E, are *estradiol* and *estrone,* which converts into *estriol.* Estradiol is the strongest-acting estrogen, and predominant in young women; estrone is weaker than estradiol, and predominant in postmenopausal women. Estriol, which is much weaker than either estradiol or estrone, is the predominant estrogen for supporting and hydrating your vulva and vagina.

As you've discovered, estrogen can have a wealth of benefits for your sexuality and health. At the same time, researchers have found that estrogen can increase your risk of certain cancers, especially in the breasts and uterus. How could something normally so beneficial play a role in such health-compromising conditions? To help answer this question, and understand more about the role of estrogen in your health, it's worth looking at why cancer happens.

Although the ultimate causes may be mysterious, many researchers agree that a person who gets cancer has an immune system that isn't working as well as it should. Your body produces cancer cells every day, but the powerful surveillance system of your immune cells renders them harmless and unable to multiply and turn into cancerous conditions. This is why you can help prevent cancer with everything you discovered earlier in this book about keeping your immune system in peak form.

Some authorities on the subject of hormones and cancer—including Jonathan Wright, M.D., who helped popularize bioidentical hormones—believe that estrogen doesn't cause cancer but can act as fuel to a fire if the cancer is estrogen-sensitive. On the other hand, if taking hormones makes you healthier by improving your sleep and your ability to cope with stress, it may help keep your immune system strong, resilient, and able to ward off any type of cancer. And in recent years research has shown that estriol, which is safer than estradiol and estrone, has protective effects against breast cancer.

Your decision as to whether to use bioidentical estrogen, and how much to use, should depend on your individual situation and needs; it's best to see a doctor who specializes in prescribing it. For some patients with menopausal symptoms, I prescribe only estriol, in doses that may vary, depending on symptoms, from 1.0 to 2.5 mg applied transdermally a few times a week. For others, bi-est (a standard hormone prescription consisting of 80 percent estriol and 20 percent estradiol) is recommended, with daily doses that typically vary from 1.25 to 2.5 mg, also applied transdermally. (See Appendix F for information on transdermal hormone applications.)

— **Natural bioidentical progesterone.** In this chapter we've enumerated the many sexual and health benefits you derive from your body's natural progesterone production. As you approach midlife, with a decrease in your natural progesterone production, you may experience fewer of these benefits, and you may gain from taking natural bioidentical progesterone. And at midlife, when your ovaries stop producing hormones and your adrenal glands take over the job, it can give your adrenal glands much-needed support.

Inadequate progesterone can exacerbate many symptoms associated with menopause. In addition to diminished libido, you may experience aggravated breast tenderness and swelling, and increased water retention and bloating. In the years leading up to menopause, your symptoms may include increased PMS and menstrual cramps, heavier periods, and insomnia and anxiety during the second half of your menstrual cycles.

If you take natural bioidentical progesterone, you want to begin with a very low dose and gradually build up to the level that works well for you. Taking too much progesterone can have side effects that include nausea, headaches, dizziness, and sleepiness the morning after you take it. As with estrogen, the amount you need, and how long you should take it, depends on many factors and your individual situation. For best results, see a qualified health professional experienced in prescribing natural bioidentical hormones.

For treating exaggerated PMS symptoms in the years leading up to menopause, the recommended dose of natural progesterone is generally between 25 and 100 mg, applied transdermally each night before bed during the second half of your cycle. But if you're also taking estrogen, make sure you take at least 50 mg of progesterone a day—important to help protect you from abnormal cell changes in the endometrial tissue in your uterus. Back in the 1970s, women who took estrogen without also taking progesterone had a much higher incidence of endometrial cancer. Subsequent research found that when estrogen is taken with progesterone—more in alignment with the balance nature intended—this risk is appreciably reduced. There's no clinical justification for using estrogen without progesterone, unless for some reason a woman doesn't tolerate progesterone.

If your uterus has been removed, taking progesterone can still markedly improve your quality of life by providing you with its many libido- and health-enhancing effects. Many medical doctors tend to think that if you've had a hysterectomy, you simply no longer need progesterone—as if its sole purpose is to prevent endometrial buildup in the uterus. Again, if you need to take hormones, it's important to find a physician who specializes in prescribing them.

— **Natural bioidentical DHEA.** The libido-boosting, health-enhancing effects of DHEA make it seem all the more precious when your body's natural production decreases at midlife. As explored previously in this chapter, in addition to improving your sexual functioning and supporting your entire hormonal system, it can elevate your moods, help you overcome depression, benefit your brain, and improve your bone density—a key issue for many menopausal women.

Not every woman who takes natural bioidentical hormones for midlife symptoms needs to take DHEA. For some, the right amounts of estrogen and progesterone sufficiently ease their symptoms. But for others, taking DHEA can be essential for restoring health and bolstering libido. If you have midlife symptoms and think you may need to take DHEA, your test results (from hormone testing, as described in Appendix E) and your symptoms should direct your treatment. The symptoms you're likely to experience if your body isn't making adequate DHEA are decreased sex drive, poor memory, reduced ability to tolerate stress, and low adrenal-gland function. You may also have a diminished sense of well-being, lower overall hormonal health and vitality, fatigue, and reduced bone health.

Before taking DHEA, make sure your estrogen and progesterone levels are stabilized. If you're also taking estrogen and progesterone, I recommend waiting a month after you start doing so before you begin taking DHEA. During and after midlife, many women need to take only very small doses of DHEA to experience notable libido-enhancing effects, increased energy, and better stress tolerance—for example, a daily dose of no more than 8 mg of DHEA applied to your skin as a transdermal oil or cream. (DHEA should be taken cautiously; excessive intake can have undesirable effects.) A holistically oriented practitioner can help find your ideal dose.

— **Natural bioidentical testosterone.** Some women in midlife become acutely aware of testosterone's myriad health and libido benefits when their natural levels subside. As you've seen, testosterone is indispensable to your ability to feel excited about your life—and sexually excited as well. It can also help reduce hot flashes, night sweats, and other menopausal symptoms.

If your testosterone is low in midlife, your most noticeable symptoms are apt to be diminished libido, disinterest in sex, a lack of creativity and motivation, an inability to build and maintain muscle, and frequent fatigue. As with DHEA, treating your menopausal symptoms with estrogen and progesterone may be enough, and you may never need to take testosterone. But if you have persistent symptoms that point to low testosterone and your test results (from testing as outlined in Appendix E) bear it out, you're a good candidate for testosterone treatment. For some women, taking testosterone not only helps restore their sex drive and eliminate menopausal symptoms, but also stimulates a heightened awareness of their bodies reminiscent of the hormonal awakenings of adolescence.

If you take natural bioidentical testosterone, you can expect to achieve the desired effects with a very low dose—no more than 4 mg daily, applied to your skin as a transdermal oil or cream. A qualified health professional who specializes in natural bioidentical hormone therapy can help you determine the amount you need. As you discovered earlier in this chapter, there may be benefits to taking testosterone in conjunction with other hormones; research suggests that when taken along with bioidentical estrogen and progesterone, it may decrease your breast-cancer risk. (If you're also taking estrogen and progesterone, it's best to start doing so about a month before you begin taking testosterone.)

If you use bioidentical hormones, you need to know the substantial and surprising differences between methods of taking them. Hormones, as mentioned before, can be applied as transdermal (absorbed through the skin) oils or creams, or they can be taken orally in pill form. Many conventional doctors—as well as some who claim to practice alternative medicine—prescribe only oral pills, perhaps because other methods weren't part of their education. But transdermal application is more effective and healthier because it allows hormones to be absorbed immediately into your bloodstream. If you use oral pills, after you swallow them, they're taken to your liver, where much of their hormone content is broken down before the remaining amount—only about 20 percent—reaches your target tissue. In addition to reducing your efficiency of hormone absorption, this puts undue stress on your liver, and if you're taking estrogen, increases clotting factors that can lead to strokes. Research has shown that applying estrogen transdermally is safer than taking it as an oral pill.

(To continue your exploration of how you should take bioidentical hormones, including how to best apply them to your body and other important considerations, see Appendix F.)

Foods and Supplements to Support Your Midlife Libido by Enhancing Friendly Estrogen

The extent of your menopausal symptoms, and the degree to which they affect your sexuality, can be closely related to how efficiently your body metabolizes, or breaks down, estrogen. During the years leading up to menopause, you may ovulate less regularly, which can bring about estrogen dominance. Although your overall estrogen level naturally tends to be lower at midlife than in previous years, promoting healthy estrogen metabolism is still of utmost importance in helping prevent serious conditions like breast and uterine cancer. Your estrogen metabolism is critical because it can result in either "friendly" or "unfriendly" estrogen. (For more information on how your body can convert estrogen into either friendly or unfriendly forms, see the diagram in Appendix E.)

The following foods and nutritional supplements can noticeably improve your body's ability to make friendly estrogen and eliminate unfriendly estrogen. They can help reduce menopausal symptoms if you have estrogen dominance, or experience difficult PMS, in the years leading up to midlife. For some women, these foods and supplements provide an especially valuable means of supporting hormone replacement therapy. If you're taking estrogen for menopausal symptoms, they can help decrease your risk of breast cancer—the single biggest concern for women taking estrogen at midlife. And even if you never take it, you still stand to benefit from these foods and supplements; they can help reduce your risk of breast cancer at any time in your life.

— **Seaweed.** The rich iodine content in seaweed makes it one of the best foods for boosting your friendly estrogen metabolism and supporting your breast health.

— **Cruciferous vegetables.** You can significantly improve your estrogen metabolism by choosing plenty of helpings from the cruciferous family of vegetables (for example, broccoli), because they're high in indole-3-carbinol—a potent anticancer agent that supports your body's ability to make friendly estrogen. Include the cruciferous clan at your dinner table often, preferably lightly steamed or raw (high temperatures can destroy indole-3-carbinol). As you discovered in Chapter 2, broccoli sprouts are exceptionally powerful for their cancer-fighting potential. They're also great for your friendly estrogen metabolism.

— **DIM.** Short for *diindolylmethane,* DIM is a cruciferous vegetable extract derived from indole-3-carbinol. It may have even stronger effects than eating cruciferous vegetables because of its unique ability to promote friendly estrogen metabolism, and by helping prevent estrogen from binding to your breast cells, reduce your risk of breast cancer. To give your estrogen metabolism an extra jolt of support, take 300 mg of DIM daily.

— **Calcium d-glucarate.** This compound occurs naturally in your body, and is found in many fruits and vegetables. Particularly helpful if you've had breast cancer, or are at high risk of developing breast cancer, it promotes your friendly estrogen metabolism, supports your breast health, and may inhibit growth of breast-cancer cells. Calcium d-glucarate has a strong safety record; no side effects have been reported from taking it. The recommended dose for enhancing estrogen metabolism is 1,500 mg daily.

— **Liver lipotropic formula.** Your sex-boosting cleanse outlined in Chapter 2 includes a liver lipotropic formula—a blend of herbs and nutrients that helps your liver break down toxins more effectively and also supports your friendly estrogen metabolism. To enhance your estrogen metabolism, take two capsules of liver lipotropic formula (see Appendix C) twice daily.

Conclusion: The Gift of Harmonious Hormones

You began this chapter by exploring your six key sex-enhancing hormones, and the many benefits each provides for your body, mind, and spirit—everything from moistening your vaginal tissues to kindling your capacity for compassion. As you've seen, every day of your life your magnificent hormones nourish, stabilize, stimulate, harmonize, empower, and energize your health and your libido. Since hormonal disharmony can be harmful to your health and sexual energy, this chapter has also provided you with many effective natural methods for enhancing your sexuality by restoring equilibrium if your hormones are imbalanced.

With your hormones harmonized, you're equipped to use all of the other sex-enhancing secrets you find in this book to more fully fan the flames of passion. We now turn to Part II of our journey—our in-depth investigation of a wide range of natural means you can use for additional sexual self-empowerment. In the next chapter, you'll discover a treasure trove of tools for enriching your sex life. There are many gems still to unearth; the excitement has only just begun!

NEW
DIMENSIONS

Natural Sex-Enhancing Secrets for You and Your Partner

CHAPTER 5

APHRODISIACS

Ancient and Modern Sexual Secrets

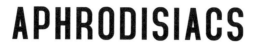

"We tend to think of the erotic as an easy, tantalizing sexual arousal. I speak of the erotic as the deepest life force."

— AUDRE LORDE, *BLACK WOMEN WRITERS AT WORK*

In this chapter, we'll explore many ways you can enhance your sexuality with natural aphrodisiacs—agents that arouse desire, intensify pleasure and erotic feelings, or otherwise stimulate your libido. Whether you currently feel the need to revitalize your sexual energy or you already have a strong libido and would like to further enhance it, the tools you'll discover in these pages can powerfully transform your sex life and boost your health at the same time.

The effects of many aphrodisiacs depend on your overall well-being; they tend to be most helpful when you're abundantly healthy. One of the underlying themes of this book—that your capacity for great health and great sex are intimately intertwined—is especially relevant when it comes to aphrodisiacs. They have a way of *proving* that great health allows you to experience states of mind and body that are otherwise inaccessible. In this sense, your health is itself a potent natural aphrodisiac.

Your greatest aphrodisiac, however, as we said in the Introduction to this book, is love. Aphrodisiacs are most effectively used in that context, rather than to enhance sexuality for its own sake.

By using them to explore new erotic landscapes, you can deepen, enrich, and enliven a love relationship. And according to some tantric teachings, expanding your capacity for erotic sensation can build another kind of love—by heightening a sense of unity with the divine.

Aphrodisiacs, after all, are named after the goddess of love. In Greek mythology, Aphrodite emerged from the foam of the sea and was carried ashore by a vulva-shaped shell. She wore a girdle with magical powers; it was believed that any woman who donned Aphrodite's girdle would arouse love in others. In Roman mythology she was identified with Venus—the goddess of love and beauty and the mother of Cupid, the god of erotic love.

Aphrodisiacs have been used by lovers worldwide since pre-historic times. As Christian Rätsch, author of *Plants of Love,* points out, archaeological evidence suggests they were used even by Neanderthal cave dwellers. Modern research has confirmed the effects of many aphrodisiacs—some contain active ingredients that induce sensations similar to those you experience when you're in love—but others may involve complex biochemical or psychological factors that elude scientific understanding. Of course, love is always unique and personal, and intimacy and pleasure highly individualistic; a sex-enhancer that works well for one couple may do less for another. To paraphrase a line written by Vatsyayana in the Kama Sutra, the classic ancient Sanskrit sex manual, the methods that lovers use to arouse each other's passion during a loving union are so mysterious as to be as indefinable as dreams.

The aphrodisiacs you'll explore in the pages ahead include some of the world's oldest and best-kept secrets for enhancing your sexuality naturally, and the most effective methods known to be safe when used appropriately. You may think of aphrodisiacs as substances taken shortly before lovemaking to ignite your sexual energy, but we'll examine them in a more inclusive sense here; some enhance your sexuality in less direct ways, yet have powerful long-term effects. You'll discover aphrodisiacs from the East and others from the West, some with ancient roots and others that are relatively new. You'll also learn about aphrodisiacs with familiar-sounding names and others you may not recognize. Many were so prized by our ancestors that they were passed down from one generation to the next for centuries, or even millennia.

You can enhance your sexuality with aphrodisiacs at any age, and they're likely to be especially effective if you're in your 30s or older. Beginning in your mid-30s, as your hormone levels subside, you may naturally experience a lessening of your libido. Perhaps you increasingly tend to sublimate your sexual energy into your career, family, or other responsibilities, and like countless other women feel you need something "extra"—some gentle, nurturing assistance—to fan the flames of passion. Why not treat yourself to some natural sex-enhancers? If not now, when?

Herbal Aphrodisiacs: Pleasure's Hidden Treasures

Herbal aphrodisiacs are the earth's medicinal gifts to your libido, and you have a cornucopia to choose from. It's surprising that many are still relatively unknown in the West—especially when you consider how successfully they've stood the test of time.

Herbal aphrodisiacs work in a wide variety of ways. Some may increase your levels of "feel-good" brain chemicals known as neurotransmitters, which can positively affect your moods, sexual vitality, and receptiveness to pleasure. In other cases, they directly affect your sexuality by stimulating nerves in your genitals, or they support your adrenal glands, lifting your libido by helping you better cope with stress. And some herbal aphrodisiacs can assist you through the stages of arousal and orgasm, or help you hold your sexual energy at a higher plateau for longer periods of time, allowing you a whole new experience of your sexuality.

Many herbal aphrodisiacs additionally boost your libido by increasing your level of nitric oxide (NO). When you have ample NO in your body, there is increased blood flow to all your tissues because it dilates your blood vessels—including those that supply your vagina and vulva. This not only enhances your sexual response, but also brings numerous health benefits to your sexual organs. In *The Secret Pleasures of Menopause,* Dr. Christiane Northrup calls NO "the spark of life," describing it as "the actual molecule that determines physical, emotional, spiritual, and sexual wellness in menopausal women (and everyone else)." The bottom line: you can give a resounding *yes* to NO.

153

As they increase your NO level, many herbal aphrodisiacs can further help recharge your sexual energy by decreasing inflammation throughout your body, stimulating your overall well-being, and accelerating your flow of chi. As you discovered earlier in this book, if your chi is stagnant or not moving freely, you're vulnerable to various physical and emotional setbacks that ultimately lower your libido.

Some of the best herbal aphrodisiacs, including some effective NO boosters, have a long history in traditional Chinese medicine. Over the course of many centuries, Chinese physicians perfected herbal formulas (blends of herbs and natural substances) renowned for their effects on libido and sexual performance. Before you use them to boost your sexual energy, however, it helps to gain some insight into their place in Chinese medicine.

Ancient Chinese physicians understood the close links between sexual energy, overall health, and what we call lifestyle choices. In the West, people sometimes perceive sexual energy as if it should always be there, but Chinese medicine teaches that your sexual health depends critically on cultivating strong chi, and that your vitality ultimately governs your libido. As previous chapters have explored, you have to make countless lifestyle choices over the course of many months and years in order to claim your health, which includes your sexual health.

Some Chinese aphrodisiacs work by not only enhancing your sexuality but also strengthening your chi, boosting your well-being, improving your immunity, helping your body heal, and potentially increasing your longevity. They may not give you immediate results, but by gradually shifting the inner "chemistry" of your health over time, they bring about long-lasting transformations in your libido. One of their secrets is that they don't work alone; the context of your lifestyle is everything. The correlation between your overall health and the effectiveness of aphrodisiacs is never so clear as with certain Chinese herbal formulas. They can significantly enhance your sexuality—but only as long as you consistently safeguard your health. With some Chinese formulas, life is fair: those who make the best lifestyle choices end up having more fun!

Another secret to many Chinese aphrodisiacs (and some non-Chinese ones, too) is balance: along with all the other factors that support your health, you need to balance your yin and yang energies. Strengthening only one or the other ultimately throws off your equilibrium, exhausts your energy, and diminishes your libido. This is why taking higher amounts of certain Chinese aphrodisiacs doesn't always mean increased sexual energy and can even have the opposite effect. Some Chinese herbal formulas support your yin energy, and some support your yang energy. Others, well known for their dualistic properties, support *both* simultaneously; they contain compounds that can, paradoxically, both relax and stimulate your nervous system.

This is especially important for your sexuality, because women typically benefit most from aphrodisiacs that are both yin and yang, taken for an extended time to gently nourish their sexual energy. (Men can benefit from these, too, but often respond well to mainly yang aphrodisiacs taken for a shorter duration to stimulate bursts of sexual energy.) As a woman, you have sexual energy that is a composite of many forces you need to balance in your life. Your sexual response requires some yang, stimulating energy, but you also need to feel yin, relaxed, receptive, loved, and loving.

Let's look at the "top 12" herbal aphrodisiacs, beginning with some Chinese classics. They aren't listed here in order of importance or effectiveness; their benefits vary from one person to the next, so you may need to experiment to discover which suit you best.

1. **Chinese ginseng.** One of the best-known herbal aphrodisiacs, Chinese ginseng (also called *Panax ginseng* or *Korean ginseng*) is legendary for its ability to increase sexual energy, stamina, and vitality. Although the herb is especially effective for men, it can enhance your sexuality, too—not as a short-term sexual stimulant but as part of an herbal formula to gradually build your libido over time. Chinese ginseng is known as a "sexual tonic" because of its long-term toning and modulating effects on your sexual chi and nervous system. It can support your libido if you feel tired, yet help you relax if you feel tense. As you found earlier in this book, it can also be warming, nurturing, and circulation-promoting for your entire pelvic region, and you can use it to treat or prevent vaginal dryness or atrophy of your vulvar and vaginal tissues.

Modern research, providing ample support for ancient findings, shows that Chinese ginseng contains compounds that can mimic your sex hormones, as well as stimulate your body to secrete hormones. It also contains *ginsenosides*—compounds that can increase your physical and mental efficiency, but without the stimulating effects of caffeine. In addition, research shows that Chinese ginseng can improve athletic performance, alleviate stress, reduce fatigue, and prevent neurological disease.

Chinese ginseng helps your body adapt to stress through its effects on your adrenal glands. An article in the journal *Medical Hypotheses* described how it affects enzymes that influence your adrenal stress response; some of these enzymes break adrenal stress hormones down into inactive compounds, and others have additional stress-relieving effects. The net result: your body has greater energy reserves—including those you need for flowing, abundant sexual chi.

Chinese ginseng is well known in Chinese medicine as a powerful herb for creating yang energy. It's usually prescribed to women combined with other herbs because it may be too yang by itself for some women to take long-term. If taken alone by menopausal women, for example, it often increases hot flashes. (On the other hand, one study found that taking the herb by itself prevented vaginal atrophy and dryness in menopausal women.)

For nourishing sexual chi, the recommended dose of Chinese ginseng for women, if taken by itself, is 200 mg, containing 7 percent ginsenosides, two to three times daily. (The dose for men is higher, as you'll see later in this book.) Avoid taking it too late in the day, which could cause insomnia, and refrain from taking it if you're pregnant or lactating, on blood-thinning medications, or have hypertension.

2. **Cordyceps.** A rare mushroom, cordyceps has been prized for at least a thousand years in Chinese medicine. It's the Shangri-la of aphrodisiacs; somehow, its wonders remained little known in the West until relatively recently. Naturopathic physicians and other alternative practitioners first began to "discover"—or rediscover—its benefits in the 1980s. Interest surged in 1993 when a group of Chinese runners broke several world records, and their coach attributed their performances in part to cordyceps.

In traditional Chinese medicine, cordyceps is considered a "potent sexual tonic." It has a unique ability to build your sexual energy over time by enhancing both your yin and yang energies, making it an ideal aphrodisiac for women. In addition to elevating libido, it's also used to increase energy and endurance, relieve fatigue, and treat sexual dysfunction. Modern research confirms that cordyceps has antioxidant properties, can improve your immunity, increases blood flow to your organs, and can help your body work more efficiently by boosting your lungs' oxygen uptake (the amount of oxygen you use) during exercise.

In Chinese medical formulas, cordyceps is often combined with other ingredients to enhance sexual response. Taken as a single herb, the recommended dose is 500 mg two to three times daily. The best type of cordyceps is the pill form; look for pills made by a hot-water extraction process that pulls out the herb's most active constituents. (See Appendix C.)

To enhance your libido and strengthen your chi, cordyceps should be taken daily for at least three to six months. The container label may recommend taking it on an empty stomach. This works for most people, but some experience mild digestive discomfort, so you may prefer taking it with food. Cordyceps is generally very safe and well tolerated, but refrain from taking it if you're nursing, pregnant, or running a fever.

3. **Rehmannia.** The root of the rehmannia plant, native to Asia, has an extensive history of medicinal and aphrodisiac use in Chinese culture. It's usually prescribed not as an individual herb but blended with other ingredients, often in herbal formulas that have aphrodisiac effects. It's a superb herb for nurturing your yin energy—particularly appropriate for female sexual energy—and creating balance if you're also taking herbs that stimulate your yang energy. Rehmannia is said to enhance your libido by drawing chi and vital energy into your sexual and reproductive organs, and is described as "food for your kidneys," with the potential to rejuvenate your energy, strengthen your chi, and increase your longevity.

Rehmannia has also traditionally been used for treating menopausal symptoms, which makes it an especially good libido-enhancer for women in midlife. Modern research hasn't

determined exactly how rehmannia works, but it appears to provide support for your adrenal glands—which, as you discovered in
Chapter 4, are crucial for your sexual energy—and help you adapt
to stress. According to some sources, rehmannia additionally contains a compound that may increase your body's production of sex
hormones.

One of the most widely used Chinese herbal formulas containing rehmannia is known as "Six Flavor Rehmannia Pills." The
typical dose is eight pellets three times daily, but recommendations vary depending on the product.

4. **Epimedium.** Even though epimedium is one of the most
powerful sex-enhancing herbs in Chinese medicine, it's unfamiliar to many in the West. Epimedium is known in Chinese medicine as *Yin Yang Huo,* which translates as "Horny Goat Weed." (Yes,
that really is the name. Legend has it that epimedium's potent
properties were discovered when Chinese goat herders observed
their flock fornicating prodigiously after grazing on a patch of the
herb.)

According to Chinese medicine, epimedium strongly influences your kidney and liver meridians—important for your sexual
chi—and fortifies your yang energy. The herb is said to "tonify
life's gate," which means that it strengthens the chi that allows
new life to be created. It's traditionally used to treat infertility in
women and impotence in men, as well as promote overall health
and longevity.

From a Western perspective, epimedium's active constituent,
icariin, can augment sexual desire by stimulating your sensory
nerves; it's believed to especially affect nerves in your genitals.
Epimedium also increases nitric oxide, thereby improving blood
flow to your sexual organs and promoting their sensitivity. It may
additionally boost your libido by supporting your adrenal glands,
and enhance your moods by increasing your serotonin and dopamine levels. Other benefits include improving and regulating
immunity, and helping lower high blood pressure.

Since epimedium is a strongly yang herb, women shouldn't
take it by itself (although men can in some cases, as you'll see in a
subsequent chapter). It's best for women if used in herbal formulas, combined with yin-supportive herbs like rehmannia, to create

a balanced effect. Avoid using epimedium regularly if you have an already overactive sex drive, a high fever, insomnia, anxiety, or hot flashes. You shouldn't use epimedium if you have low blood pressure or you're on blood-thinning medications.

5. **Reishi.** Also known as *lingzhi* in Chinese (*reishi* is the Japanese name), the reishi mushroom is one of the earliest medicines used in Asian cultures for promoting health and sexual fulfillment. Due to its ancient reputation for increasing longevity, it became known in Chinese medicine as the "mushroom of immortality." It has been widely used as an aphrodisiac, to treat infertility, and for many other sex-related benefits.

Extensive research has found that reishi contains compounds with numerous potential health-enhancing effects. It can activate your immune cells and build your immunity, support your adrenal glands, lower your cholesterol and decrease unfriendly cholesterol, and help protect your liver and promote liver detoxification. In addition, reishi has anti-inflammatory, antioxidant, and potential anticancer effects. And the list goes on: it can reduce allergic responses, help improve white-blood-cell count, support memory in older people (and may help prevent Alzheimer's disease), and decrease some side effects of radiation and chemotherapy.

The effects of reishi on your sexuality aren't as immediate as with some aphrodisiacs. You don't take it a few hours before sex to boost your libido, but long-term, over a period of months, to gradually strengthen your chi and overall vitality, and eventually intensify your sexual chi. In the terminology of traditional Chinese medicine, it stimulates not only your chi but also your "kidney essence"—a special form of chi passed down to you by previous generations and stored in your kidneys—to allow for a powerful, slow-motion transformation of your sexual energy.

The recommended daily dose is 800 to 1,200 mg, containing 14 percent polysaccharide and 4 percent triterpene.

159

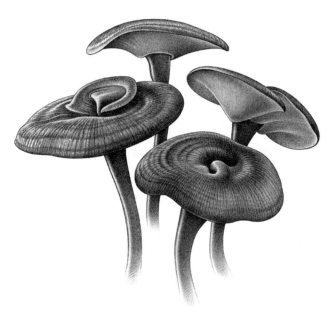

Reishi mushrooms.

6. **Ginkgo biloba.** The ginkgo biloba tree, one of Earth's oldest surviving plants, has long been considered sacred in Asia, and extracts from its leaves and seeds have been used for healing and aphrodisiac purposes since ancient times. Modern research confirms that ginkgo biloba can improve your sexual response; it appears to increase nitric oxide and enhance your sexuality by promoting blood flow to your vagina and vulva. And research indicates that ginkgo biloba, taken along with another herb that we'll explore below, can increase sexual desire, frequency of sex, sexual satisfaction, and orgasmic potential for many women.

A study published in the *Journal of Sex & Marital Therapy* found ginkgo biloba can help both women and men with sexual dysfunction occurring as a side effect of antidepressant medications. Women responded more than men, but both showed marked improvements in four phases of sexual response: desire, excitement (including increased lubrication in women and erection in men), orgasm, and resolution or "afterglow."

While ginkgo biloba is enhancing your sexuality, it's also offering you a host of other potential health gains. It can provide antioxidant benefits, thin your blood, strengthen the walls of your blood vessels, promote circulation throughout your body, and improve your memory in your senior years.

The recommended dose is 40 mg three times a day, as a standardized extract of 24 percent ginkgo flavonglycosides. Side effects are uncommon, but may include slight digestive disturbances or headaches. Avoid taking ginkgo biloba if you're pregnant or on anticoagulant medications.

7. **Catuaba.** Catuaba is well known in its native South America; songs celebrating its powers as an aphrodisiac have been sung by the Tupi Indians of Brazil for hundreds of years. Catuaba preparations, typically derived from the bark of a number of trees found in Brazil, have traditionally been used to enhance sexuality and treat decreased sexual desire due to fatigue.

Researchers have isolated a variety of active constituents in catuaba, including beneficial plant sterols, that seem to back up its historical uses. Animal studies have shown that it dilates blood vessels, so it appears likely that catuaba, like many other aphrodisiacs, has the ability to increase nitric oxide.

Catuaba is also reported to calm nervous tension and reduce anxiety, while simultaneously stimulating the brain and nervous system. With these dualistic effects—in terms of Chinese medicine, both yin (relaxing) and yang (stimulating)—it may be a particularly good herb for enhancing women's sexuality by creating balance. Catuaba also offers special benefits for men; it has been proven efficacious in treating impotence and increasing male libido. Other potential benefits for both women and men include mitigating pain, providing antiviral properties, improving memory, and treating general exhaustion.

For supporting sexual function and enhancing sexuality, the recommended dose is 500 mg once or twice daily. (Look for products from reputable companies that verify the legitimacy of the plant source.) No toxic effects of catuaba have been found to date, and it appears to be free of other side effects as well.

8. **Suma.** Also known as *Brazilian ginseng,* the root of the suma plant has been used as an aphrodisiac and sexual stimulant for centuries. It has also been a prized herbal medicine to address a wide variety of ailments and disorders; its nickname among the

indigenous people of Brazil translates as "for all"—a reference to its traditional uses for treating practically every health condition.

Suma's aphrodisiac powers, and many of its medicinal benefits, are supported by modern research. Animal studies have shown that it can increase sexual activity and potency. One study, which looked at the effects of suma and damiana, found that both boosted sexual performance, whether combined or used independently.

The active constituents in suma are plant sterols that may support hormonal balance and increase levels of estrogen and progesterone in women, and testosterone in both women and men. This makes it potentially valuable for helping smooth out the precipitous hormonal fluctuations that some women experience at midlife or during their menstrual cycles. It has been used to increase libido while also treating symptoms of both menopause and PMS.

Suma is an effective adaptogen, which means it can help restore your overall health, enhance many of your body's functions, and support your adrenal glands during stressful times. It appears to help improve, balance, and regulate the immune system as well. Suma may also have the ability to bring oxygen to cells, improve energy efficiency on a cellular level, relieve pain, decrease inflammation, and enhance athletic performance.

As an overall sexual enhancer for both women and men, the recommend dose is 500 mg once or twice daily. Because of suma's potential effects on hormone levels, it shouldn't be used by anyone who's had a hormone-driven cancer such as breast or prostate cancer.

Sex, Drugs, and . . . a Quick Fix for Women?

You may have heard that the pharmaceutical giants are seeking to develop a "Viagra for women." They certainly have a giant financial incentive; it may be just a matter of time before such a product is marketed with extravagant claims broadcast all over the media. If that happens, however, you can be sure it won't be a natural solution, and as with Viagra and other drugs, it will most likely have undesirable side effects. And the illusion that sexual enhancement can be had in a synthetic pill could deprive women of the many benefits, pleasures, and empowering feelings that come from boosting their own libidos through natural means. If you're motivated to enhance your sexuality and your health without resorting to drugs, you'll probably always prefer natural alternatives—even though a health-care system dominated by pharmaceutical corporations may have little use for them.

9. **Muira puama.** The wood of this small South American tree, often referred to as "potency wood," has been considered a highly effective medicine by many generations of healers. Muira puama has traditionally been used as an aphrodisiac and nerve stimulant; according to some sources it has also been used to increase potency, lower erotic inhibitions, and treat infertility.

A number of active compounds have been found in muira puama, although it isn't yet clear which may be responsible for its aphrodisiac effects. More research is needed, but studies appear to back up muira puama's libido-benefiting attributes. A study in 2000 at the Institute of Sexuality in France, reported in *Advances in Therapy,* looked at 202 pre- and postmenopausal women with low libido. After taking a combination of muira puama and ginkgo biloba for a month, 65 percent reported significant increases in their frequency of sexual fantasies and desires, rate of sexual intercourse, and overall satisfaction with their sex life. They also reported greater intensity of sexual desire, increased excitement associated with sexual fantasies, improved ability to reach orgasm, and elevated intensity of orgasms. Another study at the same institute found that taking muira puama on a daily basis was effective in treating 62 percent of men with low libido, and 51 percent of men with erectile dysfunction.

The recommended daily dose of muira puama for women is 500 mg, preferably taken in the morning. (The daily dose for men is typically between 500 and 1,500 mg.) If taken later in the day, its stimulating effects may cause insomnia for some people.

163

10. **Damiana.** The botanical name of this Latin American herb, *Turnera aphrodisiaca,* makes no secret of its potential effects on your sexuality. Damiana has long been used by the native people of Mexico to increase sexual energy in the pelvis, enhance fertility, and provide a wide range of other sexual benefits. It has been traditionally recommended for treating decreased sexual desire associated with what today we would call nervous-system debility.

Modern research shows that damiana contains alkaloids that improve pelvic blood flow, increase genital sensitivity, and have stimulating effects similar to caffeine. An animal study reported in *Psychopharmacology* in 1999 found damiana effective in improving sexual performance and treating impotence; the authors concluded that the results support its long-standing reputation as an aphrodisiac.

Both women and men can use damiana, but it appears to have extra benefits for women. Because it has progesterone-like effects, damiana can assist in balancing women's hormones if they have estrogen dominance, and help with infertility due to low progesterone. Other benefits may include relieving menstrual cramps, improving concentration, and helping prevent urinary tract infections.

You can drink damiana as a tea—although the taste is bitter, so it's often mixed with other herbs. For a wonderful feminine herbal aphrodisiac tea, blend equal parts of damiana, lemon balm, oat straw, and chamomile. Damiana leaf can also be taken in capsule form; the recommended dose is 450 mg up to three times daily.

11. **Maca.** In the previous chapter we explored the use of maca for treating midlife symptoms, strengthening your hormonal system, and stimulating your production of estrogen and other hormones; our focus was on its promise as an alternative to hormone replacement therapy for menopausal symptoms. Maca deserves additional attention here because of its special place in the pantheon of aphrodisiacs.

The root of the maca plant has been used for centuries in Peru to enhance sexual energy, and researchers have found a number of active compounds that may explain its effects. The aphrodisiac potential it holds for women is closely related to its effects on your hormones: it's because of maca's ability to both increase and regulate hormone production that many women who take it report increased libido. Maca can have even stronger aphrodisiac effects on men, which we'll explore later in this book.

In addition to increasing your sex drive via your hormones, maca can also help relieve stress by supporting your adrenal glands and promoting reduction of your stress-hormone level, according to a study published in *Phytotherapy Research* in June 2004. The recommended dose for women is 1,000 mg twice daily. (The dose for men is higher, as you'll discover in Chapter 7.) Research indicates maca is safe, and studies haven't reported side effects.

Over-the-Counter Herbal
Formulas as Aphrodisiacs

There are many herbal formulas on the market for enhancing your libido. Hot Plants for Her contains catuaba, maca, ashwagandha, rhodiola, and Siberian ginseng. As you've seen, catuaba is a traditional aphrodisiac, and maca can enhance your sexuality by boosting the activity of your entire hormonal system; ashwagandha, rhodiola, and Siberian ginseng can all support your libido by improving your adrenal-gland function, helping you adapt to stress, and increasing your sense of well-being.

Another herbal product, known as Women's Libido, contains blue vervain, damiana, ginger, maca, sarsaparilla, *Tribulus terrestris,* and wild oats. For supplier information on either of these products, see Appendix C.

---

12. **Yohimbine.** Derived from the bark of the yohimbe tree native to West Africa, yohimbine is a powerful sexual stimulant. Its reputation as an aphrodisiac is due to the high content of yohimbine hydrochloride in the bark's extractions. In both women and men, yohimbine increases blood flow and nerve impulses to the genitals. Research shows that it's an effective treatment for those with sexual dysfunction due to the usage of antidepressant medications such as selective serotonin reuptake inhibitors. Yohimbine acts like a strong drug, so men who need extra erection support may want to choose it over other aphrodisiacs.

Yohimbine is controversial, and not safe for everyone, because of its high potential for toxicity. It has many possible adverse effects, and shouldn't be used freely or without caution. As of this writing, yohimbine products are sold over-the-counter; you may find yohimbine under other names, including yohimbine HCl, yocon, and yohimex.

Yohimbine is also available from doctors as the prescription drug yohimbine hydrochloride. It's highly recommended that you see a doctor trained in the use of yohimbine hydrochloride and use it within safe guidelines. If you take too much of yohimbine's active ingredient, or take it along with any of the drugs known as monoamine oxidase inhibitors (MAOIs), the side effects could include nausea, vomiting, anxiety, panic attacks, headaches, and dangerously high or low blood pressure. Avoid yohimbine if you're pregnant or breast-feeding, or have liver disease, kidney disease, heart disease, high or low blood pressure, diabetes, post-traumatic stress disorder, anxiety, depression, or schizophrenia. Men with prostate problems should also avoid it.

There are important dietary restrictions to follow if you use yohimbine. Taking it along with certain herbs, or caffeinated drinks like coffee, tea, some soft drinks, maté, or guarana, could increase your risk of dangerously high blood pressure. It also shouldn't be taken along with cheese, red wine, liver, decongestants, diet aids that contain the amino acid tyramine, chocolate, sauerkraut, beer, or soy sauce.

Again, if you take yohimbine, seek professional guidance. For enhancing a woman's sexual function, the dose used by some researchers has been 6 mg daily, but it would be a good idea to start with 2 mg or less and increase to 6 mg daily only if needed. (See Chapter 7 for dosage recommendations for men.)

"Gentler" Herbs for Your Treasure Trove of Pleasure

The herbal aphrodisiacs we've explored thus far have the potential to strongly influence your sexuality in many ways. At times, you may also want herbal enhancers that work more subtly to boost your libido. The following are two of the best in this category. They can relax your energy, lift your moods, and gently coax you and your partner into pleasure. Although they're generally less intense than many other sex-enhancers in this chapter, it should be noted that they can be very individualistic in their effects; it's possible that you'll find them as stimulating as the aphrodisiacs we've explored in the preceding pages.

— **Kava kava.** The root of this plant has been used medicinally by Polynesians for thousands of years, often mixed with coconut juice. Kava kava has become popular worldwide for its ability to provide calming effects without hindering mental clarity. It can support your libido by relieving tension after a busy day, decompressing your nervous system, and allowing you to relax and get "in the mood" for sex. One effective over-the-counter product, Kava-Colada (made by Eclectic Institute) contains kava kava, dried coconut milk, and pineapple. The recommended daily dose is 600 to 1,200 mg.

Although millions of people have taken kava kava safely and without side effects, there have been some reports of liver toxicity. It appears these were due to either taking it in conjunction with pharmaceutical medications that have potential liver toxicity, or certain modern preparation methods that may result in higher toxicity. Kava kava should be taken only in appropriate doses that are properly prepared, and not in combination with prescription drugs or over-the-counter medications.

— **Ashwagandha.** The root of this South Asian plant, also known as *Indian ginseng,* has been widely used in Ayurvedic medicine for aphrodisiac and longevity-promoting purposes. Its active compounds can help increase your energy, yet at the same time facilitate your ability to sleep. Ashwagandha is a general nerve tonic with calming effects, and research shows that it can not only relieve anxiety but also treat depression. It additionally offers support for your adrenal glands, as well as anticancer, immunity-enhancing, and anti-inflammatory properties.

To use ashwagandha to boost your libido, it should be taken regularly for an extended time; it rejuvenates your sexual energy by gradually supporting your overall health. The recommended daily dose is 300 to 500 mg, standardized to contain 1.5 percent withanolides, taken in the morning.

Flower Power:
Enhancing the Mood for Great
Sex with Flower Essences

Flower essences are botanical remedies you can use to create a variety of gentle effects on your moods and emotions, such as feeling more relaxed, centered, or present in the moment. Some serve as "subtle aphrodisiacs" by helping nurture intimate emotions and release feelings that may prevent you from completely enjoying sex. The following remedies are recommended for enhancing sex by helping you get past emotional blocks you may experience. You can take them for a few days, or a few weeks; once you've made the desired emotional shift, stop taking the remedy.

— **Rock water.** Rock water is used for enhancing your libido if you feel sexually impeded by excessive self-discipline and control. It's especially recommended for those with anxiety about sexual performance because of perfectionist tendencies, and to help open a person up to new insights and sexual feelings.

— **Pine.** If you grew up in an environment filled with negative messages about sex—that it's "wrong," or not to be enjoyed—pine remedy can help liberate your emotions and release old self-defeating thoughts. It's recommended for people who, even in long-term relationships, don't allow themselves to feel pleasure—or if they do, feel guilty afterward.

— **Mimulus.** Mimulus can help you summon feelings of courage if you're experiencing ungrounded fears about sex—for example, if you feel afraid of failure or disgrace, or apprehensive around issues of performance. This flower essence can also be used for trepidation about a first sexual experience.

— **Crab apple.** Crab apple can help create healthy emotional shifts if you find sex to be somehow "unclean," or imagine that your own natural bodily functions are impure. This remedy may assist in transforming these feelings so that not only sex, but everything else in your life, becomes more enjoyable.

Stimulating Your Passion with the Essential Secrets of Sensual Scents

Scents, sensuality, and your senses are deeply connected; your sense of smell gives you a direct channel to your limbic system, the "emotional center" of your brain—critical to your capacity for sexual attraction, intimacy, and love, as you discovered in Chapter 1. By way of your olfactory nerve, scents bypass your cerebral cortex—the conscious, rational part of your mind—and reach right into your moods and feelings. This is why scents can stir strong emotions and sexual responses before you become consciously aware of them, and why a simple scent, wafting through the air, can instantly bring back a flood of passionate memories. One patient described meeting her first love after a 20-year absence: "When we embraced, I took in his scent and suddenly felt an intensely powerful emotional pull."

The speed with which scents can affect you, combined with their ability to evoke overwhelming sensual feelings, makes aromatherapy unique. Some essential oils are among the most immediate of all aphrodisiacs in their sex-enhancing effects, and for many women the most profoundly seductive. Essential oils can swiftly transform your mental and emotional landscape, shifting your awareness away from busy, analytical thoughts and creating a relaxed mood for romance and pleasure. They can expand your erotic horizons and reshape your physical responses. Using an essential oil when you have sex can "teach" your limbic system to associate that scent with pleasure, further heightening its future stimulating effects. And of course, essential oils can also enhance sex by deeply affecting your partner—and making you more alluring to him.

Scents from natural essential oils have been used as aromatherapy throughout history for their aphrodisiac potential, and many not only have eroticizing effects but also give you health benefits. Let's look at four of the most time-tested essential oils used for generating desire and pleasure:

— **Ylang-ylang.** Traditionally used as a perfume, the oil produced by ylang-ylang flowers has a rich, succulent scent and a great reputation for inducing sensual moods and erotic experiences. In Indonesia, where ylang-ylang is highly regarded as an aphrodisiac, the beautiful yellow blossoms are strewn on newlyweds' beds. Its compelling fragrance, believed to have narcotic-like effects, may also be a sexual restorative; according to some sources, it nourishes sexual chi by acting on the adrenal glands. Since it has both relaxing and uplifting qualities, ylang-ylang is sometimes recommended for dispelling feelings of anxiety about sex.

— **Jasmine.** Because its flowers bloom only during nighttime, jasmine is also known as "Queen of the Night"—a fitting moniker for a plant used since ancient times to elicit sexual desire. The essential oil extracted from the strongly scented flowers, which contains a compound similar to musk, exudes an aroma often described as intoxicatingly sweet and sensual. Its euphoric effect is created, in part, by supporting the release of "feel-good" brain chemicals such as endorphins. Jasmine essential oil can be used to increase positive feelings, foster sexual confidence, create a more sensual ambience, and rouse passion.

— **Lemon balm.** Also known as *melissa,* lemon balm is a member of the mint family, characterized by beautifully veined, heart-shaped leaves. The essential oil of this wonderful herb, often of particular benefit for women, has traditionally been used to enhance libido, elevate moods, soothe nerves, and restore inner equilibrium. (Several modern studies have shown that it can help reduce anxiety and promote sleep.) It's also recommended in aromatherapy for nurturing your emotions, opening your heart, and cultivating a greater sense of freedom to express your innermost feelings. In addition to using the essential oil on your skin, lemon balm can be taken as a tea, allowing you to ingest its oils and let them work from within. You can gently support your body, mind, and spirit by drinking a few cups of the tea daily; to make it, steep one teaspoon of the dried herb in a cup of boiling water for ten minutes, and strain.

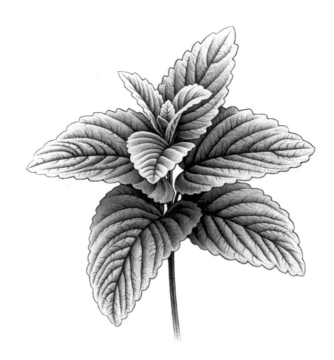

Lemon balm.

— **Sandalwood.** An ancient aphrodisiac, sandalwood has a woody scent that's both pungent and enticing. Some women and men tend to find sandalwood highly attractive, perhaps because it contains compounds similar to human pheromones—scents our bodies produce that trigger sexual responses in others (which we'll explore in the following section). Sandalwood has long been used for meditative purposes, but it's also a captivatingly erotic fragrance that seems to quiet the mind and focus sensual awareness on the here and now. It's ideal for those who become easily distracted during sex and need assistance turning their thoughts inward to the realm of sensing and feeling.

You can apply essential oils to your skin in the morning to set the mood for the day, or apply them before sex by adding them to a massage lotion or oil. You may also want to let their fragrances fill your bedroom or living space by using them in spray bottles or herbal diffusers. (Essential oils and aromatherapy diffusers are available at many specialty stores and online.) If you use them on your skin, you can apply them to intimate areas such as your inner thighs or between your breasts, but avoid your clitoris, vulva, or other mucous membranes. You can also apply essential oils to acupressure points, allowing them to penetrate your meridians and further stimulate your sexual chi. The following points are recommended: Kidney 27, Kidney 1, and San Jiao 4. (To locate these points, see Appendix A.)

Sex-Messaging:
The Aphrodisiac Potential of Your Secret Scents

Your nose serves as a kind of sexual sextant—a finely tuned instrument for navigating your erotic environment—and gathers far more information than scientists once believed possible. The study of human pheromones is still in its infancy; there's much we don't know, and much to discover. The current state of research can perhaps be summed up by saying *no one knows what your nose knows*. But there's been some fascinating research in recent years. Whether you emit pheromones in the same sense as some animals do, and precisely what sexual signals you send and detect, isn't yet entirely clear. However, it would be difficult to imagine a more fantastic (and potentially romantic) picture than the one that seems to be emerging from the world of biological research on human pheromones. The following is an interpretive overview.

You have an invisible "scent cloud" emanating from your body at all times, released from your breath and perspiration on your skin, drifting through the air around you like an aura. These scents are believed to be produced mainly in special glands concentrated in your underarms, genitals, anus, chest, abdomen, breasts, and naval. Your scents contain important chemical signals—personal information about you that's instantly detected by anyone you meet, allowing that person to "perceive" your scent-essence. At the same time, it's a two-way exchange; you're picking up on similar personal information about the other individual.

But there's a delightful catch: neither of you is conscious of all the information you detect; much of it is perceived subliminally rather than through your normal sense of smell. In a sense, you're using a subtle form of communication hidden from both of you (which is why we use the term *secret scents*), yet it can affect your individual moods and behaviors. It may cause each of you to have intuitions about the other—you may feel attracted, repelled, or indifferent—without any conscious awareness of what's passing between you. This may go a long way toward explaining the proverbial "woman's intuition," or the "sixth sense." And what we call love at first sight may often be a matter of love at first scent.

Further complicating this marvelous picture, your secret scents are uniquely blended with your body's other natural scents—the ones you *are* conscious of—because the two are released in unison. For example, a man's secret scents are typically released in conjunction with a consciously recognizable, musky "male" scent. Thus, you and the other person each have a distinct "scent print" or "scent identity" that announces who you are to the world.

Your secret scents may affect the men in your life in more ways than are currently known. During your teenage years, your body begins sending secret *sexual* scents into your environment. The ones you release as a woman are distinct from those emitted by men, and each gender reacts differently to the secret sexual signals from the opposite sex. Research indicates that your secret sexual scents can cause a rise in the production of a man's hormones, which may have direct effects on his body, such as increased rate of facial-hair growth. And when you ovulate, you emit secret scents that are especially attractive to men.

By the same token, over the course of your life you're affected in countless ways by men's secret sexual scents. Research suggests that girls consistently in the presence of male sexual scents may enter puberty sooner than other girls. Not only can a man's secret scents attract you and enhance your sexual arousal, but they have the greatest effects when you're ovulating; if you're exposed to a man's secret scents combined with a musky scent, it can cause you to do so sooner than you might otherwise. If you're in the presence of a man's secret sexual scents on a regular basis, the length of your menstrual cycles may be shorter and more consistent.

Research shows that your secret sexual scents also affect other women. It appears that they can cause a phenomenon you may have experienced—the synchronization of menstrual cycles in women who spend lots of time together. Surprisingly, if you're in the presence of other women's secret scents for a period of three to four months, it may significantly increase your likelihood of sexual activity with men (more than a sixfold increase, according to one study).

You can think of your secret sexual scents as your "personal" aphrodisiacs; their sex-enhancing power is specific to you, because your scent print is as unique as your fingerprint. Since secret scents are so individualistic, human-pheromone products that purport to enhance sexuality seem limited in their potential. There's no shortage of fragrances and other products on the market—and claims that they'll make you irresistible—but evidence for their effectiveness is often all too scanty. Some contain pheromone-like chemicals synthesized in laboratories and patented. Manufacturers sometimes don't disclose ingredients, making it impossible to assess if they're natural or have the potential to cause side effects or allergies.

The beauty of your secret sexual scents is that you can't prevent their release or mask them with scents that are consciously recognized by your normal sense of smell. They're detectable regardless of perfumes and colognes—no matter how pleasant or striking—or any unpleasant body odor. All you can do is be yourself and let their hidden magic happen. You may increase their effects by avoiding unnecessary antiperspirants, or (when possible) wearing garments that don't cover your underarms or abdomen. And since the consciously recognizable portion of your scents is part of your scent print, you might want to minimize deodorants—an easy way to keep your natural essence readily detectable to your partner's "extrasensual perception."

Nutritional Aphrodisiacs: Super-Sex Supplements and Foods

If you consistently take the nutritional supplements and follow the Great Sex Diet outlined in Chapter 2, all of the nutrients and foods you consume will bolster your libido. In addition, certain supplements and foods can pack an extra punch of pleasure potential. First, let's look at two nutritional supplements that merit special mention for their unique ability to stimulate your sexuality:

— **L-arginine.** An amino acid that's essential for your body to function optimally, L-arginine can also be an effective natural sex-enhancer for both women and men. (We'll look at its benefits for men later in this book.) It works by increasing nitric oxide and promoting blood flow to your sexual organs. L-arginine is often taken in supplement form, but it can also increase your sexual response if applied topically to your genitals, which is why it's found in many stimulating arousal creams.

A study published in the *Archives of Sexual Behavior* in 2002 found that 6,000 mg of L-arginine as a dietary supplement (along with 6 mg of yohimbine) notably increased female sexual response. Other research suggests that L-arginine can boost libido by working synergistically with herbal aphrodisiacs and other ingredients. A study at the University of Hawaii, reported in 2001 in the *Journal of Sex & Marital Therapy,* showed that over 70 percent of women who took the product ArginMax For Women—which contains L-arginine, ginseng, ginkgo biloba, damiana, vitamins, and minerals—experienced increased sexual desire, higher frequency of sex and orgasm, enhanced clitoral sensation, decreased vaginal dryness, and improved overall sexual satisfaction, with no significant side effects.

L-arginine is found in many foods, including nuts, beans, fish, eggs, chicken, and chocolate, but for full aphrodisiac benefits it's best taken as a supplement; recommended doses are generally between 2,000 and 6,000 mg daily. One of L-arginine's added benefits is treating hypertension, so if you have low blood pressure, refrain from taking it as a supplement (although it's still safe to use topically). Those with herpes shouldn't take L-arginine, or use it topically. Avoid taking L-arginine if you have a gastric ulcer, liver disease, or kidney disease.

— **PEA.** The acronym for *phenylethylamine*, PEA is sometimes referred to as the "love supplement," or the "romance chemical." As a stimulant and mood elevator, it can induce sensations of euphoria—and it's naturally released by your brain when you're in love. PEA promotes an increase in the neurotransmitter dopamine, which enhances feelings of well-being, joy, and pleasure, and can assist in treating depression.

If you'd like to elevate your PEA level, you have some attractive options: have an orgasm every day (PEA is released by your brain whenever you reach orgasm); exercise regularly (a study published in the *British Journal of Sports Medicine* in 2001 found that exercise increases PEA—one reason why exercise can improve moods and relieve depression); or eat chocolate, a rich source of PEA (see the following page).

Another way to increase your PEA level is to take it in the form of supplements derived from blue-green algae. This is more efficient than eating chocolate, and free of fat and sugar. In addition to boosting feelings of pleasure, intimacy, and well-being, PEA can also help you cope with the mood changes of PMS and menopause. The recommended daily dose is 30 to 100 mg. (Avoid larger amounts, which could cause overstimulation, insomnia, or anxiety.) PEA shouldn't be taken by nursing or pregnant women, or anyone taking MAOI medications.

Along with these supplements, some foods have gained special status as sexual victuals, with the potential to give you an added dose of libido nourishment. All of the "super-libido foods" you explored in Chapter 2 provide extra support for your sexual health in a general way, but those in this category are known, or reputed, to provide nutrients that specifically stimulate your sexuality.

Although people have searched for foods with sex-enhancing powers since the dawn of history, some long assumed to be aphrodisiacs may owe their reputations to placebo effects—which might make them interesting food for thought, or food for fantasy, but not true aphrodisiacs in the biochemical sense. (On the other hand, it may be that their active constituents haven't yet been discovered.) Let's take a look at some foods believed to have aphrodisiac powers, and how each qualifies as erotic fodder:

— **Sweet potatoes.** Including sweet potatoes in your diet can support your sexuality because they're especially high in vitamin B_5—important for your adrenal-gland health, which promotes production of your sex hormones. As a source of carbohydrates, low-glycemic sweet potatoes are also preferable to white potatoes, which have a higher glycemic index. (As you saw in Chapter 2, low-glycemic carbohydrates are healthier than ones higher on the glycemic index.) Sweet potatoes are a perfect complement to meals, and they also make great snacks for great sex.

— **Chocolate.** The flagship food aphrodisiac, chocolate is chock-full of love-conducive, pro-pleasure ingredients. (No wonder so many people choose chocolate for Valentine's Day gifts.) Not only does it contain both PEA and L-arginine, but also the compound theobromine, which according to some sources has aphrodisiac potential and stimulates the central nervous system. Eating chocolate can be a sensual experience, and it's also high in antioxidants that support your immune system and help fight free radicals. Dark chocolate is best—as pure and unsweetened as possible. The extra fat and calories in some chocolate products can have long-term unhealthy consequences and anti-aphrodisiac effects.

— **Oysters.** The reputed aphrodisiac prowess of the sexy mollusk may be largely a credit to its suggestive shape, although oysters also provide a wealth of minerals that can indirectly support your sexuality by boosting your overall health. They're extremely high in zinc (helpful for both female and male sex-hormone production, and particularly important for male sexuality, as you'll discover later in this book), and a rich source of vitamins and beneficial omega-3 fats.

— **Pomegranates.** Historically, pomegranates have been associated with love, eroticism, and fertility (perhaps because of their copious seeds), and believed by traditional cultures to have aphrodisiac or medicinal properties. Although no specific aphrodisiac ingredients have yet been isolated in these large berries, research shows they're high in antioxidants and other healthy compounds. Pomegranates offer special support for men's sexual issues, but they can also promote your general sexual well-being with potential benefits that include improved circulation, reduced blood pressure, and enhanced cardiovascular health.

— **Chili peppers.** Chili peppers can undoubtedly make you feel hot, but they may not necessarily elevate passion to a fever pitch, as some anecdotal reports suggest. It appears that their effects vary widely from one person to the next, so their aphrodisiac potential could be a matter of individual reaction. Your mouth feels like it's aflame when you eat chili peppers because they contain *capsaicin,* a chemical that stimulates your skin sensitivity, accelerates your metabolism, increases your heart rate, and energizes you. You may have heard claims that kissing your partner shortly after chewing a chili pepper can transfer the stimulating effects to his mouth, but it's not recommended. The heightened sensitivity that capsaicin causes in skin and mucous membranes is unpredictable, and painful for some people.

— **Honey.** Although some native cultures have long believed that honey enhances sexuality, a chemical agent with specific aphrodisiac properties hasn't yet been found in it. In addition to sugars, some types of honey contain beneficial vitamins, minerals, enzymes, amino acids, and other ingredients. If you consume honey, remember that it's high in sugar; use it in moderation to keep your blood-sugar level stable—a plus for your long-term health and sexuality.

Minimizing *Anti*-Aphrodisiacs in Your Diet

A few dietary options deserve special attention for their potential to seriously hamper your long-term sexual health. It's fine to indulge in these on occasion, but if you consume them regularly they may eventually catch up with you, zap your health, and create a lot of zeros for *eros*.

— **Alcohol.** Alcohol is often associated with sex because of its inhibition-reducing effects. This may promote the misleading view that decreasing your awareness with alcohol will somehow improve your sexuality. (In fact, too much alcohol lowers your sexual response and dulls your perception of pleasure, and alcohol can also negatively affect your sex hormones.) More important, alcohol is a known toxin with addictive properties. As you discovered in Chapter 2, you can dramatically enhance your sexuality by *de*toxing—not by "toxing" (or intoxicating). Like some other drugs, in the short run alcohol may make you feel invulnerable, but in the long run its numerous health consequences can deprive you of many of the joys of a vibrant sex life.

— **Fatty foods.** You generally want to avoid fatty foods because over the long haul they congest your liver, which can make you feel tired, heavy, lethargic, and decidedly unsexy. Of course, fatty foods also promote weight gain, which isn't especially favorable to your overall health and libido either. The Great Sex Diet in Chapter 2 will help you steer clear of fatty foods.

— **Sugar.** Excessive sugar intake may not only be detrimental to your sexual energy by causing your blood-sugar level to become disrupted, but may also reduce your ability to become aroused by increasing your body's production of the stress hormone cortisol. In addition, it can compromise your production of DHEA, your pro-libido "sexy hormone."

— **Caffeine.** Consuming too much caffeine can break down testosterone (as you've seen, vital to your libido) and make PMS symptoms more likely.

Conclusion: Keeping Your Natural Aphrodisiacs in Perspective

You've explored a varied range of natural sex-enhancers in this chapter, from herbal aphrodisiacs to flower essences, essential oils, hidden sexual scents, and nutritional tips and treasures. Some of these aphrodisiacs and enhancers are, in a sense, your natural inheritance—closely guarded secrets that were passed down to you by many generations of your ancestors. All of them can be invaluable for transforming your sexuality at any time in your life.

Whenever you use aphrodisiacs and sex-enhancers, keep in mind that their effects tend to depend on your sexual health as a whole and your total state of well-being. As you turn the page to begin a new chapter in your journey—our survey of another, more extensive category of passion-promoters and libido-lifters— remember that all aphrodisiacs and sex-enhancers are more apt to be effective if you use them in combination with everything else you've discovered in this book.

CHAPTER 6

ACCENTUATING SENSUALITY

Other Sexual Secrets with Aphrodisiac Potential

"It is the soul's duty to be loyal to its own desires."

— REBECCA WEST, QUOTED IN A. L. ROWSE'S *GLIMPSES OF THE GREAT*

Like many people, when you hear the word *aphrodisiac,* you probably think in terms of lotions, potions, pills, herbs, oils, aromas, nutrients, or supplements. All of the aphrodisiacs we've explored in the preceding chapter fit into these categories. By some broader definitions, however, the term may be used to encompass many other kinds of tools and techniques you can use to arouse desire, intensify erotic feelings, incite passion, or otherwise magnify your pleasure potential.

In this chapter, we'll peruse pleasure-enhancers in this wider sense—an eclectic category that includes Western and Eastern approaches, embraces modern and ancient means, and ranges from down-to-earth practical solutions to mind-expanding methods of amplifying and stretching your capacity for erotic sensation. We'll take a close look at stimulating lubricants, techniques for increasing the flow of chi to your genitals, special libido-elevating devices and procedures, tantric practices, and more. Whether any of these tools and techniques qualify as aphrodisiacs in the conventional sense may be a matter of academic opinion. In any event, many of them can certainly have aphrodisiac-like qualities, and you may find that their effects unquestionably establish them as major sex-boosters.

As with conventional aphrodisiacs, the sex-enhancers in this category are likely to be most effective when you have abundant health—for example, if you've applied the techniques in Chapter 1 for maximizing your mental and spiritual well-being, as well as the other lifestyle recommendations in Chapter 2. Your health itself, as we pointed out in Chapter 5, can be a potent aphrodisiac.

At the same time, the pleasure facilitators we'll explore in this chapter, like the aphrodisiacs in the previous chapter, can help to transform your sex life regardless of whether you currently feel a need to recharge your sexual energy or you already have a robust libido and would like to further stimulate it. Either way, the tools and techniques you'll discover in the pages ahead have the potential to play an important role in enhancing your sexual health and libido.

Sexual Lubricants and Stimulants

As we shift our focus to sexual lubricants of all kinds, it's worth noting that this group of enhancers dovetails perfectly with the category of aphrodisiacs we've explored thus far. Any of the enhancers in the preceding chapter, by stimulating your libido, can increase your need for sexual lubricants.

In turn, the sexual lubricants you use can further promote your pleasure in a variety of ways. Some serve as gentle enhancers and "indirect aphrodisiacs" by moistening your vaginal and vulvar tissues, mimicking and multiplying the effects of your body's own natural lubrication and allowing you to have sex that feels relatively friction-free. There are lots of lovely lubricants in this group to choose from.

Another class of sexual lubricants can be described as "extrasensual enhancers"— agents that can induce arousal and augment sexual pleasure. These act as aphrodisiacs in a more direct way. They simulate the effects of your body's natural lubrication while at the same time further stimulating pleasure through other means; this ability to simultaneously simulate and stimulate makes them unique among pleasure-enhancers.

Any sexual lubricant you use should be as natural and healthy as possible, because the receptive mucous membranes of your vagina and vulva can easily absorb their ingredients into your body. Examine their ingredients as carefully as the foods you eat; some products presented as natural and healthy include synthetic or toxic compounds that could undermine your health. Many synthetic lubricants contain chemicals first designed for use on automobiles or in oven cleaners, so it's no surprise that some women experience unpleasant reactions. The following is a short list of ingredients to *avoid* putting on your sensitive genital tissues:

— **Parabens.** Parabens are synthetic preservatives that can be absorbed through your skin. They can mimic estrogen in your body, and may be linked to increased risk of breast cancer.

— **Petroleum or petroleum-derived ingredients.** Whenever possible, refrain from using products with petroleum-based ingredients, including multipurpose lubricants like Vaseline petroleum jelly, on your genitals. They may contain impurities linked to cancer and other health conditions; they can also coat your skin, impeding its normal functions and not allowing it to "breathe."

— **Silicone oils.** Silicone oils may have toxic side effects, and as with petroleum-based products, they may coat your skin, affecting its normal functions and permeability. Silicone can have many names on product labels, including *dimethicone, highly polymerized methyl polysilozane, methyl polysiloxane, mirasil DM 20,* and *viscasil 5M.*

— **Phenoxyethanol.** At high concentrations, phenoxyethanol can be harmful if absorbed through your skin, cause reproductive damage, and according to the FDA, depress the central nervous system in newborns. The breakdown of phenoxyethanol in your body releases phenol, which can adversely affect your immune system. The Environmental Working Group (EWG), a nonprofit research organization, lists phenoxyethanol as a moderate hazard, with possible links to toxicity and skin irritation. Although it's found in very low concentrations in some sexual lubricants, you'd do best to keep away from it—especially when many products without it are available.

— **Glycerin and glucose.** As sugars, glycerin and glucose may feed *candida,* a yeast that's normally present in small amounts in the healthy vagina, but which can proliferate and cause vaginal yeast infections in women prone to them.

— **Propylene glycol.** Propylene glycol may cause burning or tissue irritation in some women. Astroglide, a common over-the-counter lubricant, contains this ingredient.

— **Chlorhexidine.** An ingredient in some multipurpose lubricants, such as K-Y jelly, chlorhexidine can be irritating to some women.

Even if you haven't had problems with synthetic lubricants, using natural products can make a difference in your sex life. In the pages that follow you'll explore some lubricants we've found, both moistening and extra-stimulating, that claim to be more or less natural, and we'll compare their pros and cons. Not all are recommended; as you'll discover, some contain ingredients you may want to avoid. Manufacturers sometimes change ingredients in their products—some lubricants that seem appealing now could later became problematic, or vice versa—so you need to stay vigilant and make sure the products you use remain beneficial. (And refrain from using anything if you are allergic to any of its ingredients, or your partner is, or if it causes either of you any discomfort.)

Sex-Facilitating Lubricants

The lubricants in this group not only facilitate sex by replicating the effects of your body's natural lubrication—most have a distinctly "slippery" quality conducive to pleasurable sex—but many also hydrate your vulvar and vaginal tissues, which can provide additional long-term benefits for your sexual health. (However, you can enhance pleasure by using sexual lubricants regardless of whether you need to relieve vaginal dryness.)

— **Aloe Cadabra.** This delightful, primarily organic lubricant contains 95 percent aloe vera gel, which makes it both an effective sexual lubricant and, if used on a daily basis, helpful for keeping your vulvar and vaginal tissues well nourished, healthy, and moisturized. It also contains vitamin E oil, xanthan (a natural food-grade gum), citric acid, trace amounts of potassium sorbate (a natural food-grade preservative), and sodium benzoate (another common food preservative). Aloe Cadabra is water based, latex-friendly, and available in three blends: Natural Aloe, Tahitian Vanilla, and French Lavender.

— **Firefly Organics Intimate Botanical Moisturizing Crème.** An exceptional all-natural sexual lubricant made with food-grade plant ingredients, this product by Applied Organics contains sunflower-seed extract, canola-seed extract, cocoa butter, beeswax, shea butter, and vitamin E. It's an emollient (it softens and soothes skin), has moisturizing properties, nourishes a woman's delicate genital tissues, and can help with midlife vaginal dryness. It's even waterproof (in case you plan to have underwater sex). The only drawback may be that it's incompatible with latex condoms.

— **Sliquid Organics Natural (water based).** The ingredients in this effective latex-friendly lubricant are water; plant cellulose from cotton; aloe; vitamin E; cyamopsis (guar conditioner); potassium sorbate; citric acid; and extracts of hibiscus, flax, alfalfa, green tea, and sunflower seed. The company also makes a lubricant called Organics Silk, but a number of its ingredients are listed by the EWG as potentially problematic, so this product is preferable.

Great Sex and Latex

We include "latex-friendly" as a criterion for a good sexual lubricant because condoms are commonly made of latex, but many people are unaware that some sexual lubricants can dissolve it, causing condoms to break apart during sex. Water-based lubricants are latex-friendly; oil-based lubricants aren't. Whether you use latex condoms for safe sex (see Appendix G) or birth control (see Appendix H), it's important to use latex-compatible lubricants.

— **Yes Oil-Based Organic Lubricant.** This hypoallergenic lubricant is pH compatible with your own vaginal tissues, beneficial for your skin (so there's no need to wash it off), and nonstaining. Its plant-based ingredients include organic cocoa butter, organic shea butter, two organic emollient oils (almond and sunflower oil), organic beeswax, and vitamin E. This is another good lubricant that's not compatible with latex condoms.

— **Yes Water-Based Organic Lubricant.** It's unfortunate that Yes Water-Based Organic Lubricant, which is latex-friendly, contains phenoxyethanol (although its concentration is below one percent), because its other ingredients would make it a good choice: organic aloe, organic flax extract, three plant-based gums (guar, locust bean, and xanthan), citric acid, and potassium sorbate.

— **Sylk Personal Lubricant.** Sylk Personal Lubricant, which has a pH of 4.7 (the approximate average pH of a woman's vagina for most of the month), contains purified water, kiwi extract, vegetable glycerin, sodium citrate, xanthan gum, citric acid, potassium sorbate, citrus-seed extract, and grapefruit-seed extract (a possible skin irritant for some women). As mentioned earlier in this chapter, the glycerin may pose a problem; however, this is an all-natural, latex-friendly lubricant with no chemical additives or artificial preservatives.

> ## Sex-Enhancing Household Lubricants
>
> In a pinch—maybe the mood is just right, and your passion can't wait—you may have several lubricants among the oils right in your pantry that can enhance sex or relieve vaginal dryness: olive oil, coconut oil, and cocoa butter are especially effective; and almond oil, vegetable oil, and other natural oils can also be used (although none are latex-friendly). Steer clear of egg whites or honey, even though they're natural; egg whites can set off acute vaginal infections, and honey may cause vaginal yeast infections in women prone to them.

— **Higher Nature V Gel Sexual Lubricant.** This nonstaining lubricant, safe if swallowed, is produced by Elixir Health. It contains organic aloe; purified water; glycerin; panthenol; kelgin (seaweed); comfrey; marigold; vitamins A, D, and E; zinc citrate; potassium sorbate; and the food-grade preservative sodium benzoate. As noted above, the glycerin may be of concern to some women, but otherwise this is an effective latex-friendly lubricant.

— **Good Clean Love Almost Naked Personal Lubricant.** This lubricant seems healthy at first glance; it contains water, agar (seaweed), aloe-leaf juice, xanthan gum, lemon citrus, and vanilla fruit. However, it also contains lactoperoxidase (a synthetic enzyme), glycerin and glucose (which, as you've seen, may both be problematic for some women), benzoic acid (listed by the EWG as a moderate hazard with possible links to toxicity and skin irritation), and glucose oxidase. Since this product includes ingredients that may not be right for everyone, you might want to exercise some caution when using it.

	Aloe Cadabra	Firefly Organics Intimate Botanical Moisturizing Crème	Sliquid Organics Natural (Water Based)	Yes Oil-Based Organic Lubricant	Yes Water-Based Organic Lubricant	Sylk Personal Lubricant	Higher Nature V Gel Sexual Lubricant	Good Clean Love Almost Naked Lubricant
Organic ingredients?	95% or greater	95% or greater	Partly (5 ingredients)	95% or greater	95% or greater	No	Partly (1 ingredient)	95% or greater
Free of potentially problematic ingredients?	Yes	Yes	Yes	Yes	No	No	No	No
Water based?	Yes	No	Yes	No	Yes	Yes	Yes	Yes
Latex-friendly?	Yes	No	Yes	No	Yes	Yes	Yes	Yes
Contains animal products?	No	Beeswax only	No	Beeswax only	No	No	No	No
Tested on animals?	No	No	No	No	No	No	No	No

Edible Lubricants

If you want the freedom to ingest your lubricants without worrying about their health effects, there are plenty of natural options available. Here are some edible lubricants you might find suitable to your taste. (Note: Only the last is latex-friendly.)

— **Honey Girl Organics Personal Lubricant.** Made in Hawaii, this pure, simple lubricant can be used not only during sex but also at other times to keep your vulvar and vaginal tissues hydrated. It contains organic extra-virgin olive oil, water, organic beeswax, vitamin E, organic pollen, and organic propolis.

— **Devour Me Lickable Oil.** This line of oils, made with sweet almond oil, is available in flavors that include Piña Colada, Strawberry Kiss, Cherries Jubilee, Chocolate Mint, and Crème Brûlée.

— **Love Balm by Sensuous Beauty.** This ingestible balm is made from coconut oil; vitamin E oil; and essential oils of lavender, bergamot, and myrrh. Its long-lasting slippery sensation also makes it a good choice for full-body massages.

— Hathor Aphrodisia Lubricant Lickeurs. Available in a variety of flavors—including Coconut Orange, Chocolate Strawberry, and Hazelnut Caramel—these organic, luscious lubricants contain no honey or glycerin (they're stevia sweetened), so they don't increase risk of yeast infections. The other ingredients are water, vegetable propylene glycol (which, as noted, may be irritating to some women), organic flavorings, acacia gum, vitamin C, jujube zizyphus, Siberian ginseng, and epimedium.

Extra-Stimulating Lubricants, Gels, and Creams

Unlike the lubricants we've explored thus far, these lubricants, lotions, gels, and creams have additional built-in pleasure-promoting properties. Some provide all the benefits of moistening lubricants, but go one step further by including ingredients designed to give you a "pleasure-plus" experience. Of all types of sexual enhancers and aphrodisiacs, these are among the most immediate in their effects. They can be gently massaged directly onto your clitoris and surrounding vulva before or during sex, and they may achieve the desired effect within minutes, or even seconds.

Many stimulating lubricants contain ingredients like niacin and L-arginine that enhance arousal by promoting blood flow to your delicate clitoral and vulvar tissues. Some contain other ingredients, such as cinnamon, which increases blood flow while also creating "warming" sensations, or menthol and peppermint, which have "warming yet cooling" effects. If you have untreated VAD, or any inflammation in your vaginal area, there's a chance that some of these stimulating ingredients could be irritating. (And if you have genital herpes, L-arginine could make you more prone to outbreaks.)

All too often, stimulating lubricants, gels, and creams contain chemicals you'll want to avoid. Let's look at the pros and cons of some products on the market, and consider which are the most natural and safest for your sensitive genital tissues:

— Zestra. A female arousal oil shown in studies to enhance sexual response, Zestra can also help provide moisture to your vulva and vagina. It contains borage-seed oil and evening-primrose oil, herbal extracts of angelica (known in Chinese medicine

189

to increase circulation and flow of chi) and coleus forskholii (a smooth muscle relaxant), vitamins C and E, and theobromine (a chocolate-derived ingredient that may be a key to Zestra's effectiveness). Zestra is available over-the-counter at many drugstores, but is not compatible with latex condoms.

— **Vigorelle.** A high-quality natural enhancement gel, Vigorelle is edible, pH balanced, and latex-compatible. It has a minty smell, an olive squalene base, and a consistency similar to your body's own natural lubrication. The ingredients include L-arginine; ginkgo biloba; wild yam; damiana; suma; peppermint; tea-tree oil; vitamins A, C, and E; hyaluronic acid; aloe; shea butter; and apricot-kernel oil. It also contains vegetable glycerin, which in some women could increase the potential for vaginal yeast (although the tea-tree oil might help prevent this), and a small amount of grapefruit-seed extract, which in sensitive women could be irritating. This product's prohibitive price may be its biggest drawback.

— **Blossom Organics Pure Pleasure Arousal Gel.** This water-based, latex-friendly gel contains barbadensis-leaf extract, hydroxyethyl cellulose, sorbitol, L-arginine, niacin, organic rose-hip oils, evening primrose, menthol, herbal extracts of peony and passionflower, and glycerin (which could contribute to yeast infections in susceptible women). The company also carries a warming oil that's glycerin- and L-arginine-free—although not latex-friendly—containing many of the above ingredients in a base of sunflower, borage-seed, and linseed oils.

— **Sliquid Organics Sensation.** An effective latex-compatible stimulating gel, Sliquid can also help soothe and hydrate your vaginal tissues. The ingredients include water; plant cellulose; aloe; vitamin E; guar conditioners; extracts of hibiscus, flax, alfalfa, green tea, and sunflower seed; menthol; potassium sorbate; and citric acid. (This company also makes a nonstimulating lubricant, Sliquid Organics Silk, that contains the silicone product dimethicone—not recommended for your vulva or vagina.)

— **Oh! Warming Lubricant.** This stimulating gel by Emerita may seem healthy, but on closer inspection contains some ingredients of concern: propylene glycol (as previously indicated, a potential irritant), glycerin (which may increase likelihood of yeast infections in susceptible women), and honey (another yeast-infection concern). Its other ingredients include cinnamon, hydroxypropyl cellulose (an emulsifier, fairly benign in low doses), and lactic acid (rated as a moderate hazard by the EWG, and a possible skin irritant for some women). This product may be particularly irritating if you have VAD or your vaginal tissues are sensitive due to low estrogen during midlife. Despite the potential drawbacks, however, some women regularly use this product without problems and find it effective.

— **Response Topical Sexual Arousal Cream.** This is another Emerita product that looks good at first glance but includes a few ingredients you may want to avoid: glycerin (again, a potential problem for some women), sucrose (a sugar that can increase likelihood of yeast infections in susceptible women), and phenoxyethanol, which as you've seen may pose problems. It also contains rosemary, cinnamon, menthol, niacin, amino acids, and other natural ingredients.

— **Valentra.** This mostly natural, water-based, condom-friendly cream unfortunately contains dimethicone, a silicone-based compound rated by the EWG as a moderate hazard with possible links to toxicity, and which some data suggest shouldn't be used long-term on your delicate genital tissues. It also contains vegetable glycerin, which could increase the potential for vaginal infections in some women. Other ingredients include L-arginine, vegetable squalene, wild yam, organic aloe, gotu kola, ginseng, damiana, Saint-John's-wort, soy lecithin, vitamins A and D_3, peppermint oil, and organic oils of rose hip and evening primrose.

— **Intimate Organics.** Although this company offers a number of products that appear healthy and environmentally friendly—they're made with many organic ingredients, are 100 percent vegan, and are free of many undesirable chemicals—they also contain phenoxyethanol and a few other potentially problematic ingredients.

191

Enhancing Sex with Erotic Stimulators

Research suggests that more than half of women use vibrators for sexual stimulation at some time in their lives. If you decide you want to do so, there are all kinds of options on the market to explore—from sleek to multipurpose, and from remote-controlled to waterproof. There are devices specifically designed to stimulate your G-spot, and others conceived for your clitoris. Some women may find that G-spot-stimulating vibrators increase their ability to experience ejaculatory orgasms, as described earlier in this book.

One company that offers a variety of vibrators you may find appealing is Natural Contours Intimate Massagers. If you're interested in a more inventive twist, consider the Better Than Chocolate OhMiBod waterproof wireless music vibrator, which connects with your iPod to vibrate in sync with your favorite music (and to the tune of about $100). If you're in the market for something much more exclusive, there's the Yva—an 18-karat gold designer vibrator by the Swedish company Lelo, with a $1,500 price tag.

The Sex-Enhancing Power of Vaginal Strengtheners and Releasers

The next category of sensual enhancers that we'll explore includes unique devices and methods you can use to increase your capacity for pleasure—and magnify the effects of any other type of sex-enhancer or aphrodisiac. As enhancers and aphrodisiacs go, the tools and techniques in this category could be considered "sleepers." You might not *expect* them to impact your sexuality . . . only to be amazed by how much they have to offer. They have a way of sneaking up on your libido, turning it around, and transforming it from top to bottom.

As you discovered in Chapter 3, your "hammock" of pelvic muscles, known collectively as your PC muscle, supports your sexual organs and contributes to your sexual pleasure; when you reach orgasm, it contracts with rhythmic intensity. You also discovered that you can help create stronger, more pleasurable orgasms by strengthening your PC muscle with Kegel exercises.

In addition to Kegels, and sex itself (which also increases your PC-muscle strength), some valuable ancient and modern methods can further develop, tone, and release your PC-muscle power. Let's explore how you can use them to increase your pleasure potential.

Ben Wa Balls: Ancient Secrets, Modern Methods

The exercises we call Kegels can be thought of as descendants of techniques that have been used for millennia. The ancient Chinese used weighted devices known as *Ben Wa balls,* inserted in the vagina, for training the pelvic muscles—a system of vaginal weight lifting, if you will, to increase a woman's sexual ecstasy, as well as her partner's.

Traditional Ben Wa balls, which may trace back as far as A.D. 500, consist of rounded weights of various sizes (typically between a half inch and one inch in diameter). They've been referred to as *vagina balls, pleasure balls,* and more recently, *Kegel balls.* Modern Ben Wa balls may be made of metal, jade, plastic, rubber, or other materials. Jade, prized for thousands of years in China, is an especially appropriate material for Ben Wa balls; according to traditional Chinese Medicine, it can help build your feminine yin chi, as well as release stuck chi and negative sexual feelings, in your vagina and pelvis.

Ben Wa balls can be solid or hollow, and some contain movable internal parts, including devices that vibrate. They're often paired, with a string connecting them. There are many variations of Ben Wa balls available online, including Duotone balls and Smart balls, which both tend to be larger than traditional Ben Wa balls and consist of hollow balls with smaller balls inside them; the small ones bounce rhythmically inside you with each motion of your body, creating vibrating sensations that some women find highly pleasurable. These balls may make strengthening your PC muscle an extremely enjoyable experience.

With Ben Wa balls, you can take your Kegel exercises to a whole new level, using a variety of balls to strengthen and tone your vaginal walls and inner pelvic muscles. With regular use, some women experience noticeable increases in vaginal lubrication, vaginal and clitoral sensation, and orgasmic pleasure. Ben Wa balls are effective because they give you a focal point that helps you become aware of whether you're squeezing your PC muscle; at the same time, they require you to keep your PC muscle firmly tightened to hold them in place as you move around.

The first time you use Ben Wa balls, you'll want to be at home and begin with lightweight, larger balls. Empty your bladder, and use a small amount of lubrication on the balls if needed to insert them. Stand with one foot on a chair and gently insert them into your vagina with your finger. It should feel approximately like using a tampon. Try wearing the balls for an hour a day, then work up to longer periods of time over the course of a few weeks. In the early going, you'll find it easier to hold the balls in place while sitting or standing with your legs together. When your PC muscle grows stronger, you'll be able to stand with your legs apart, and eventually try the advanced technique of squatting. (Some women reach the point where they can even wear them exercising.) As you develop increasing PC strength, you'll also be able to gradually increase the weight of the balls.

To remove Ben Wa balls, relax your PC muscle, bear down on your pelvis as if you're coughing or having a bowel movement (squatting helps), reach your finger into your vagina, and pull them out. Some Ben Wa balls have a string attached for easy removal. (I recommend this type; one patient was unable to remove them on her own.) After each use, wash them well with warm soapy water.

Ben Wa balls shouldn't be used if you have severe bladder or uterine prolapse (your bladder, or uterus and cervix, is extending down into your vaginal opening), you're pregnant, it has been less than six weeks since you've given birth and you had incisions that haven't healed, it has been less than six weeks since you've had vaginal surgery, you have a vaginal infection, or you have cervical or uterine cancer.

Vaginal Cones: Modern Secrets, Modern Methods

Another effective way to increase your capacity for pleasure, become familiar with your PC muscle, and develop its strength is with specialized weighted cones held in your vagina. Vaginal cones have numerous benefits: in addition to enhanced sexual response and erotic sensation, women who use them report improved libido, more energy, and less anxiety. They're especially helpful for building your "resting" muscle tone—you don't want your PC muscle too lax while at rest—and preventing and treating urinary incontinence. Vaginal cones also help prevent prolapse of the bladder or uterus, and PC muscle weakness after childbirth or menopause.

To begin using vaginal cones, wear a larger, lighter cone for one to five minutes twice daily. This helps you become aware of the cone while squeezing your PC muscle to hold it in place. Once you're accustomed to wearing it and you've begun to build PC-muscle strength, you can progress to smaller, heavier cones, which require more flexing to hold in, and eventually work up to wearing heavier cones for 20 minutes twice daily. (Some types of cones may allow you to increase the weight without changing the size.) Listen to your body, and gradually lengthen the time that you wear each cone. Once you've mastered the technique, you can wear cones while going about your daily activities; for an extra challenge, apply enough lubricant to a cone to require greater flexing to keep it in place. Wash your cones with soap and water after each use.

It's generally recommended that you wear vaginal cones daily over an 8- to 12-week period. For many women, this is a sufficient course of therapy to develop noticeable improvements in PC-muscle strength and pleasure during sex; others wear cones longer to obtain the desired results. You shouldn't use vaginal cones if you have severe bladder or uterine prolapse, or any other conditions previously described that would preclude the use of Ben Wa balls. Vaginal cones are usually sold in sets containing cones of various sizes and weights. For information on purchasing them, see: **www.medgo.com** or **www.kegelme.com**.

195

Enhancing Your Sexuality with "Acu-pleasure"

Acupressure may not be an aphrodisiac per se, but it can certainly boost your sexual energy. For added effects, you can use it in combination with any sex-enhancer in this chapter, or any aphrodisiac in the preceding one. The following points are recommended for increasing your sexual energy, nourishing your sexual organs, and improving the flow of chi that courses through them: *Kidney 27, Ren 15, Ren 17, Large Intestine 4, San Jiao 5, Pericardium 6, Heart 3,* and *Heart 7.* To strengthen your sexual chi, press firmly on these points for a few minutes each day. To locate them, see Appendix A.

Pelvic and Vaginal Self-Massage with Acupressure

You can also enhance your capacity for pleasure with pelvic and vaginal self-massage in conjunction with acupressure. Massage stimulates your circulation, brings blood and nutrients to your tissues, releases tension, and literally helps you get in touch with your body; acupressure, as noted in the accompanying sidebar, can support your chi and your sexual energy. Their combined effects can increase your sexual vitality regardless of the condition of your PC muscle, but their benefits may be especially pronounced if it has become chronically tight.

Like many women, you may have a tight PC muscle without realizing it. This can have many causes, including consistently poor posture or body mechanics, stress, giving birth, pelvic surgery, childhood injuries, pelvic trauma, or painful sexual experiences. If your PC muscle is chronically tight, no matter how much you strengthen it with Ben Wa balls and vaginal cones, you may still be unable to fully manifest your potential for sexual pleasure. Some women with this condition have decreased sexual sensation, are subject to a variety of pelvic-health issues, and feel disconnected from their sexuality. In more extreme cases, they may have chronic PC-muscle spasms, or *vaginismus* (painful contractions of the vagina), making sex difficult or impossible.

The benefits you stand to gain from pelvic and vaginal self-massage combined with acupressure—by relieving chronic PC-muscle tightness and allowing your pleasure to unfold more freely—are reflected in the teachings of Chinese medicine, which sees a chronically tight PC muscle in terms of stuck chi, or trapped energy, in your pelvis. Both massage and acupressure can help move your chi, liberating your energy for healthier, more pleasurable pelvic experiences.

Let's look at how you can increase your capacity for pleasure—whether or not your PC muscle is chronically tight—with do-it-yourself treatments. Before getting started, familiarize yourself with the abdominal acupressure points in Appendix A. You'll need a handheld mirror and massage oil, such as almond or coconut oil.

To begin, remove your clothes and lie in bed on your back, with pillows under your head and knees. Apply oil to both hands, and massage in circular strokes, gradually covering the area from your upper abdomen to your mons pubis, the soft "mound" where your pubic hair begins. Your abdominal and PC muscles are attached by connective tissues, so this can relieve tension in both. Note: Throughout this treatment, your massage technique should remain gentle, and you should feel comfortable, relaxed, and safe; refrain from touching any area if it causes discomfort. If you feel any tension or tenderness, breathe deeply, and consciously allow your tissues to relax.

Once you feel that your abdominal muscles are relaxed (this could take a few minutes), you're ready for acupressure. Press the following points, holding each for five deep breaths, or about 30 seconds: Kidney 16, Ren 6, Ren 5, Ren 4, and Ren 3. You can press two points simultaneously, one with each hand.

After you've pressed each of these points, massage your hips as you did your abdomen until they, too, feel relaxed. Then roll onto your side, place the pillow between your knees so your thighs are a few inches apart, and massage your inner thighs for a few minutes. When they feel relaxed, roll onto your back and put the pillow under your knees.

Next, massage the areas where your inner thighs meet your vulva, then massage your perineum—the area between your vagina and anus. The tissue of your perineum is helpful for gauging the condition of your PC muscle, and massaging it can both relax it and relieve PC-muscle tension. (When a woman prepares for childbirth, the perineum can be stretched and made ready with massage.) Using the mirror, locate the center of your perineum, midpoint between your lower vaginal opening and your anus. This is an important acupressure point, Conception Vessel 1 (not shown in Appendix A)—also known as "meeting of yin," because your body's yin energy converges here. By pressing on it, you can release stuck chi, nourish your sexual chi, and enhance your sexual energy. Press on this point for five deep breaths, or about 30 seconds.

With your acupressure treatment now complete, gently massage your outer labia for a few minutes, then lightly caress your inner labia. Use the mirror to locate your urethra (just above your vaginal opening); you'll want to avoid massaging it because it's sensitive to touch. Feel the tissues of your vaginal opening, and if you're comfortable exploring your vagina, use your finger (well lubricated) to carefully massage the tissues on both sides of your inner vaginal walls. If you discover any tight "ropey" areas, ever so gently massage them, breathe deeply, and focus your mind on releasing tension; you may notice they gradually become softer and more relaxed.

When you feel ready to finish your massage, slowly remove your finger from your vagina and massage upward toward your abdomen. Complete your treatment as you began, with a few minutes of abdominal massage. By re-massaging your abdomen after you've relaxed your hips, thighs, perineum, vulva, and vagina, you can further relax your abdomen and PC muscle.

If you do this treatment often, you may intuitively develop your own ways of creating greater relaxation. You may also feel empowered by becoming more intimately aware of your pelvic and vaginal tissues. Many women are unfamiliar with this part of their bodies; some touch their vaginas only for sex and bathing, but never in a therapeutic way. (The only time their vaginas may be touched therapeutically is during doctor visits.) Establishing a relationship with your pelvis and vagina in which *you* are your own healer can be a transformative experience; with such a vital, sacred part of your body, claiming your right to self-nurturance is especially important.

For further reading on pelvic self-massage, see Appendix C. If you experience chronic pelvic pain and need professional guidance with pelvic massage, some physical therapists specializing in women's pelvic health provide hands-on release techniques for the pelvis and PC muscle.

Are Your Issues in Your Tissues?

If you have any sexual issues—especially issues related to past sexual experiences that were unwanted or traumatic—loving touch to your vulva and vagina may help transform and restore your sexual health. According to some schools of thought, such as Rolfing, your bodily tissues can "remember" trauma that may have occurred many years ago, and past pain can be healed by physically and energetically releasing your tissues with massage and other techniques. In some ways, this parallels the Reichian theory that pent-up sexual or psychological energy can create "body armor"—real physical tensions and blockages in muscles and organs—that you can overcome through healthy sexual release.

Sex-Expanding Tantric Techniques: The Apex of Great Sex?

In this chapter we've explored a plethora of pleasure-enhancers in a variety of categories. There's one form of sex enhancement, however, that stands in a category all its own . . . tantric sexual practices. Although they don't involve ingestible chemical agents, tantric practices may be considered aphrodisiacs in a general sense: they're sometimes ranked among the most effective approaches to enhancing sexuality, and can unquestionably broaden your erotic horizons and multiply your pleasure potential many times over. The roots of the Sanskrit word *tantra* have links to the words *weave* and *stretch*. We include tantric sexual practices here because they allow you to weave entirely new erotic experiences, and stretch the limits of your capacity for sexual sensation.

You don't have to join an obscure sect and follow a guru to benefit from ancient tantric sexual secrets; it's easier than you might think to use them on your own (enhance sex *sans* sects) and incorporate them into your erotic life. Tantric practices may not be for everyone, but if you're in a trusting, committed relationship, and you want to explore other dimensions of your sexuality and experience a new level of intimacy, they may be right for you.

Before we explore how you and your partner can use tantric sexual practices, let's look at what they have to offer you and some key concepts behind them, based on interpretations of some tantric teachings:

199

— **Transformative sex.** Tantric sexual practices give you a refreshing alternative to sex as a brief, momentary pleasure—especially if you tend to perceive your sexuality in functional terms, as a straightforward performance with orgasm always the objective. For too many couples, sex is the typical five- to ten-minute animalistic gyration that usually culminates with male, and sometimes female, orgasm. (It's estimated that 79 percent of men, but only 29 percent of women, reach orgasm during sex.) Tantric practices can expand your sexual landscape by alleviating a man's pressure to climax quickly, vastly transforming your possibilities for pleasure, sex, and orgasm.

— **Freedom from goal-oriented sex.** Central to many tantric sexual practices is an idea that's difficult for some to grasp because it challenges fundamental notions about sexuality—that the purpose of sex isn't necessarily orgasm. In some tantric teachings, the principle of delayed gratification is taken to extremes: the longer climax is postponed, the greater the potential benefits. Goal-free sex can last for hours—as long as you and your partner choose—because the journey is the destination, and the focus is on crystallizing your awareness at every step along the way.

— **Getting beyond ego-based sex.** Another concept integral to some tantric teachings is that sex can be a way of releasing control of your ego-centered mind and becoming more conscious of pure sensation. It can be challenging for some people to surrender ego control and trust the outcome—it may trigger feelings of vulnerability and defenselessness—but the potential rewards are many: greater intimacy, trust, well-being, and inner peace, and a sense that you're not a separate entity from your partner . . . or indeed from all of life.

— **The gifts of salubrious sex.** Tantric sexual practices can open your being to healing powers that may otherwise lie dormant—by extending the length of time you have sex (thereby multiplying some of the health benefits of sex we explored earlier in this book), and allowing for greater stimulation of your sexual chi (according to Chinese medicine, a potent therapeutic force, as we touched on in Chapter 3). And on another level, tantric practices may also be deeply healing and nurturing in and of themselves, by giving you access to transformative physical and spiritual states.

— **Sacred sexuality.** The idea that sex can be a liberating, mystical experience is essential to some traditional tantric teachings. Sex isn't just about your physical pleasure—it's perceived as a way of stimulating your spiritual awareness, transcending your personal limitations, and discovering your connection to ultimate creative forces. (One tantric practitioner describes it as "finding out that at your core you're inseparable from the essence of the universe, which is pure love.") As a result, the act of sex is elevated to the highest order of spiritual importance; it can be a holy rite, and a profound sacrament. And in turn, the effects some tantric practices may have on your emotions and states of mind can instill a lasting sense of awe for the mysteries of sex.

— **Deeper bonding.** Tantric sexual practices can be thought of as a dance you and your partner perform together, a mutual meditation in motion—and at times, as you'll see, in motionlessness—that makes you much more closely connected. As a natural consequence, you're likely to experience greater intimacy, both sexually and otherwise, and discover new realms of sharing in your relationship. The importance of communication in tantric practices, for example, which we'll explore below, has a delightful way of spilling over into every other aspect of your relationship and improving your interactions in all areas.

With all of these potential gains, it's a wonder more couples don't use tantric sexual practices regularly. Perhaps the cultural tendency to compartmentalize sex—as if it's just another task to fit into your busy schedule—is partly to blame for this. In our fast-paced, goal-oriented society, tantric sexual practices seem anomalous; you have to create enough time in your life to make their many benefits possible.

There are numerous approaches to traditional tantric practices. Some involve elaborate preparatory rituals, preliminary breathing techniques, and other methods to help prime you physically and mentally for sexual intimacy. Sensual massage can be important; according to some tantric teachings, your vulva is like a flower that gradually opens and blossoms in response to loving touch. Foreplay may be deliberately prolonged to heighten your and your partner's erotic awareness prior to intercourse.

Once sex begins, the secret to many tantric practices lies in abstaining from, or delaying, the immediate pleasure of thrusting to orgasm. For instance, it's sometimes recommended that you and your partner hold a motionless embrace, with his penis in your vagina, for an extended time. Other means of enhancing pleasure may be pursued, but since orgasm isn't the goal—and resisting orgasm creates the desired effect—anything that might precipitate either partner's climax is discouraged.

Many basic tantric sexual teachings can be summed up approximately like this: Once you or your partner are close to climax, hesitate; let pleasure subside, then gradually rebuild the excitement until you're again on the verge of orgasm, and again hold off. Repeat this cycle multiple times, each time driving as close as you both can to the precipice and backing down just before either of you is swept over the edge. Eventually you'll reach the point where you're both so perfectly poised on the brink of orgasm that you won't need to move a muscle to back down; simply remaining motionless will be pure ecstasy (a word derived, fittingly, from the same root as *stasis*, or motionlessness). Stay in this state as long as you possibly can; the longer you remain on the cusp, the more profound the potential sexual and spiritual effects.

For some people, the state of prolonged near-orgasm is experienced as a kind of perpetual climax; the pleasure normally felt in condensed form as a momentary orgasm may seem miraculously drawn out in slow motion over a much longer period of time. Your sensations may become increasingly intense, allowing you to reach ever-loftier plateaus of pleasure. Some people may experience trancelike states of mind-altering euphoria. If and when orgasm eventually happens, it's usually described as . . . well, *indescribable.*

Tantric practices may be especially beneficial if you often climax at a different pace from that of your partner. As noted earlier in this book, a woman's sexual energy tends to be like a large pot on a small flame; it takes a while to warm up, but stays hot for a long time. A man's tends to be like a small pot on a big flame; it heats quickly, but doesn't stay hot as long. Once "heated up," a woman can keep simmering with multiple orgasms, but a man typically needs to cool down with a postorgasm refractory period before he can have another erection. If you and your partner want to synchronize your sexual tempos, tantric practices can be a great equalizer, allowing you to make sex last long enough to experience simultaneous peak bliss.

In addition, according to some tantric teachings a man can not only dramatically expand his ability to remain in a sexually heightened state, but also learn to climax without ejaculation and experience multiple orgasms. Some insist this is biologically possible; others believe it's a metaphorical way of describing an experience that seems to transcend any other form of sexual ecstasy, and a degree of pleasure beyond measure.

Verbal communication between you and your partner can be crucial in tantric sexual practices; some teachings recommend sex in a face-to-face sitting position to facilitate clear dialogue. In extreme states of ecstasy, with every sensation intensely magnified, words may be your best tools for holding orgasm at bay. Only through the subtle nuances of language can you give each other precise feedback on how close to orgasm you are, when you're ready for more (or less) stimulation, exactly where to touch or refrain from touching, and just how firmly or feather-lightly to caress. For giving spur-of-the-moment cues on your proximity to climax, you and your partner may want to create your own system of signals beforehand—for example, a scale of 1 to 10, with 1 being low arousal and 10 the verge of orgasm.

Sharpening your verbal sex skills can have spinoff benefits in other sexual areas. If you've become accustomed to silent sex—and often hope he'll read your mind and touch you differently—it can open up new dimensions during your non-tantric lovemaking. And with clear communication you can also steer your partner through intricate foreplay rituals that without words would be impossible. For instance, you can guide him in giving you a massage similar to the one recommended in the preceding section for pelvic and vaginal self-massage, but with an erotic slant.

Breathing techniques during intercourse are also important in some tantric sexual teachings. If you and your partner reach a transcendent state of motionless pleasure, in which even the slightest movement can trigger orgasm-like sensations, your breathing may be the only motion that either of you makes. In this state, breathing becomes an art form. One method is to alternate your breaths: when you inhale, he exhales; and vice versa. Another is to synchronize your breathing so you inhale and exhale in rhythm. (Since women usually take shallower breaths than men, he may need to match his breathing with yours.) Experimenting with breathing techniques may help you stay connected with your partner, prolong ecstasy, promote relaxation, and provide a meditative way of focusing your attention on your bodies.

Sex and Tantra: The Tantalizing (or Not) Possibilities

Tantra may be less sex-centric than you think, depending on how you define it. There are various definitions, but the term generally refers to practices based on beliefs outlined in certain Hindu or Buddhist texts. A core conviction underlying many tantric practices is that the world we perceive, including our bodies, is a microcosmic manifestation of divine creative energy. Tantric practitioners use ritualistic techniques in an effort to reach higher spiritual states by balancing and channeling this energy in their bodies.

Although in the West we associate tantra with sex, many traditional tantric rituals don't involve sex, but focus instead on meditation and adherence to rules of moral conduct. When sexual practices are involved, they're seen as a catalyst for creating experiences of mystical ecstasy that differ from sexual pleasure in the usual sense and may not involve orgasm.

With popularization in the West, tantra, like yoga, is sometimes simplified in ways that might make it seem almost unrecognizable in its native context. Just as many who practice yoga have no idea of its original significance in the theistic tradition of Hinduism (as a practice emphasizing the renunciation of bodily and mental activity), some proponents of tantra may be unaware of its original cultural roots. You can find a wide range of information about tantra online—along with plenty of hyperbole, exaggerated claims of sexual feats, and links to pornography. Despite this oversexualization, and although tantra may never become as acceptable and accessible as yoga, it similarly has a lot to offer Westerners.

Conclusion: Sex Enhancement in Perspective

You've delved into a diversity of pleasure-promoting tools and techniques in this chapter, from modern to ancient means; from Western to Eastern approaches; and from practical, down-to-earth tips to lofty, mind-expanding practices for heightening your capacity for pleasure. You've explored sexual lubricants and stimulants, vaginal strengtheners and releasers, tantric techniques, and more. In some cases, as with many of the aphrodisiacs in Chapter 5, these pleasure-enhancers have been handed down to you by many preceding generations.

Although some of the enhancers you've discovered in this chapter may not be considered aphrodisiacs in the traditional sense, all can have aphrodisiac-like qualities and be invaluable for your sexuality, whether you use them separately or in combination. As you turn to the next chapter on our voyage—the exploration of sexuality in a relationship, and the myriad ways your sexual well-being is influenced by your partner's sexual health—keep in mind that, as we said in the Introduction to this book, nothing has greater aphrodisiac potential than love.

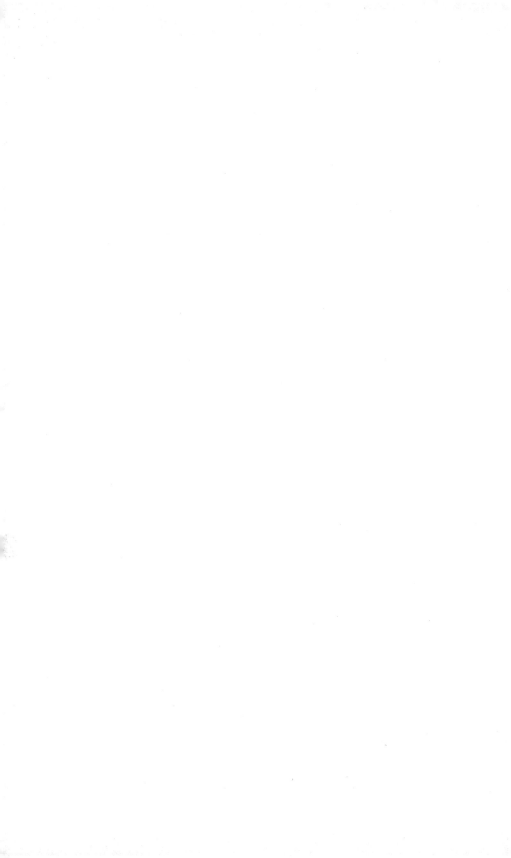

CHAPTER 7

MALE
SEXUALITY
How Your Partner's Sexual Health Affects You

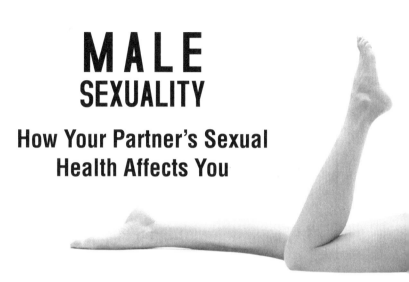

*"When we try to pick out anything by itself,
we find it hitched to everything else in the universe."*

— JOHN MUIR, *MY FIRST SUMMER IN THE SIERRA*

As a woman, you know that love, intimacy, and sex are all about relationship and partnership. You may feel, at times, that you and your partner are each a part of one another, as surely as the word *part* is a part of the word *partners*. Successful partners, by definition, are joined together, complement each other, share deeply, and in some sense complete one another.

During an intimate relationship, your sexual health and your partner's merge, with your two sexual energies closely united. If his libido is healthy, it can benefit your own immeasurably. As you've seen, your sexual energy flourishes in the presence of healthy male sexuality. The "secret" sexual scents his body releases, which you detect unconsciously, can affect when you ovulate, and over time regulate the length of your menstrual cycles.

With his sexual health in top form, you also stand to gain from the potential health benefits of sex itself: decreased stress; better circulation; enhanced moods through the release of "feel-good" endorphins and oxytocin; reduced blood pressure and greater calmness; improved vaginal lubrication; strengthened immunity; diminished pain (including pain from menstrual cramping); and lower likelihood of urinary incontinence, heart attacks, and endometriosis. On the other hand, if his libido is out of balance, it can affect yours in countless ways.

Just as your partner's sexual well-being promotes your own, so too can his overall health shape yours. If he's thriving in body, mind, and spirit, you're more likely to be in that state as well, but if his health is compromised, it can have numerous repercussions for *you*. In a sense, your two immune systems become joined at the hip; they uphold one another, for better or for worse, in sickness and in health.

In a long-term intimate relationship, enhancing your partner's health and sexual well-being enhances yours, and vice versa; vitality is reciprocity, sexuality is mutuality, and sensuality is cosensuality. And as Chapter 1 touched on, health and sexual well-being can also be of great consequence psychologically and emotionally, with the potential to affect every aspect of your relationship.

The idea that sexual partners physically and spiritually complement and complete one another was well known to practitioners of ancient Chinese medicine, which was built on the balance of opposites: feminine and masculine, water and fire, darkness and light, inwardness and outwardness, yin and yang. Sexuality is viewed as the dance between feminine inward-receptive yin "water" and masculine outward-projecting yang "fire." If you've achieved a truly balanced partnership, you and your partner can be seen as two halves of one whole, each intimately affecting the other and in close harmony, like the two interlocking shapes of the yin/yang symbol.

In previous chapters we've compared the yin, cool tendencies of female sexual energy to a large pot on a small flame (it warms slowly, but stays hot for a long time), and the yang, hot tendencies of male sexual energy to a small pot on a large flame (it heats quickly, but doesn't stay hot as long). You can use many of the tools and techniques you've discovered, including herbal aphrodisiacs with yin or yang effects, to help balance you and your partner's energies. For some couples, the tantric practices in the previous chapter can be especially helpful in synchronizing their sexual tempos. And simply being aware of the differences between women's and men's yin and yang sexual energies brings you closer, strengthens your relationship, and generally engenders harmony between genders.

This chapter will empower you and your partner with tools for enhancing his sexual health, and thereby your own. (Of course, you want to improve the health of the man you love because you care about his well-being, not simply to benefit yourself, but since this is a book for women, we're adopting a gynocentric perspective.) Women are often concerned about issues affecting the sexual health of their partner, but find a shortage of information to answer their questions. Male sexual-health needs are sometimes overlooked, perhaps because men are reluctant to discuss personal sexual matters or see doctors—statistics show the vast majority of health-care consumers are women—and as a result even some medical practitioners aren't well informed about men's sexual issues.

In the pages ahead, we'll explore the most effective ways your partner can enhance his sexuality with natural methods. Since many men have conditions that require added support, we'll also provide natural solutions to the sexual-health challenges your partner is most likely to face, including common conditions associated with lowered sex drive and function. As you'll discover, there's a lot he can do to treat or prevent these conditions—with results that can bring inestimable benefits to your shared sexuality.

Promoting Pleasure:
Male Libido Enhancement and Support

Sexual well-being can be vital to a man's health and longevity. A ten-year British study found that men having two or more orgasms a week have 50 percent lower mortality risk than men having orgasms less than once a month. According to Barry Komisaruk, Carlos Beyer-Flores, and Beverly Whipple, authors of *The Science of Orgasm,* research shows that "higher frequency of ejaculations over the years is correlated with a lower incidence of prostate cancer"—perhaps partly because fluid released from a man's prostate gland at orgasm helps clear it of potential cancer-causing substances. Frequent orgasms may also improve circulation through this sensitive area of his body, increase immune-system function, and promote health and relaxation through peak releases of oxytocin.

Whether your partner has a healthy libido and wants to further enhance it, or has low sexual energy and wants to boost it, there are plenty of options he can pursue. First and foremost, his sexuality depends on his lifestyle: all components of the sex-supportive lifestyle you discovered earlier in this book apply to him as well. This makes it convenient for you to make those changes together, incorporating them into your lives as a couple. And as you enhance your libidos in tandem, you may be surprised to find that the changes you make *more* than double the fireworks between you.

In addition, there are steps your partner can take that apply specifically to men. (Some men are averse to self-help and feel they don't need sexual enhancers. To convince your partner to consider taking these steps, it will help to approach the subject with sensitivity, and explain the benefits for both his sexuality and his health. You may also want to frame it in the context of a sexual-health plan that you implement together.) Let's begin by exploring the most effective herbs, supplements, and foods he can use to support and enhance his sexuality; later in this chapter, you'll discover that he can also use many of these for treating conditions like erectile dysfunction or low testosterone.

Herbal Aphrodisiacs for Men

Since your greatest natural aphrodisiac is love, you and your partner may not feel the need for any other form of sexual enhancement. Your attraction to each other, coupled with all of your daily physical and psychological foreplay, may be all you ever need for great sex. Or to put it differently, in a loving relationship your partner's ultimate natural aphrodisiac may be *you*. But if he ever wants to further stimulate his libido, there are some wonderful herbal aphrodisiacs that can enhance his sexuality.

A man can use many of the herbal aphrodisiacs in Chapter 5 to improve his sexual energy, including cordyceps, catuaba, suma, muira puama, damiana, kava kava, and ashwagandha. (For dosage and recommendations, refer to the descriptions in that chapter; men's doses are the same as those for women, except where noted.) Let's look at herbal aphrodisiacs that deserve extra attention because of their particular benefits for male sexuality:

— **Chinese ginseng.** Chinese ginseng, which we've explored as an aphrodisiac for women, has been used to enhance male sexual function for centuries in Asia. Modern research confirms its effects on male sexuality. Human studies show it can increase libido and improve sperm count, as well as sperm motility, and animal studies show that it can increase sexual activity and performance. In addition, research shows it can provide antioxidant benefits and help boost athletic performance, improve physical and mental efficiency, relieve stress, decrease fatigue, and prevent neurological disease.

In terms of traditional Chinese medicine, Chinese ginseng is a yang herb, recommended for a man who needs to increase his yang energy. Symptoms of yang deficiency include muscular weakness, cold hands and feet, and lower-back pain. The recommended dose for men is 500 to 1,000 mg, containing 7 percent ginsenosides, two to three times daily. It shouldn't be taken too late in the day (it could cause insomnia), or by men who are on blood-thinning medications or have hypertension.

211

— **Tongkat ali.** The aphrodisiac properties of this flowering plant, which has been used for hundreds of years in Southeast Asia to stimulate male sexuality, have been validated by modern research. Both human and animal studies show that it can reduce erectile dysfunction by promoting blood flow to the penis, and also increase testosterone levels. (Tongkat ali is considered a phytoandrogen—a plant with male hormone–like actions.) Research has additionally found that it can decrease body fat and increase muscle mass and strength in older men, and has antianxiety effects.

The active constituent in tongkat ali has been patented and sold in the United States as LJ100. The typical daily dose is one to two 50 mg pills, but some men need only one pill every other day to achieve the desired effects. In excess, LJ100 can cause aggressive moods, irritability, and insomnia.

— **Epimedium.** In Chinese medicine epimedium (also known as Horny Goat Weed, as mentioned in Chapter 5) is considered a strong "sexual tonic," traditionally recommended for treating male impotence and for a wide range of other health benefits. Icariin, its active compound, can enhance a man's libido by stimulating his sensory nerves, particularly in his genitals—definitely earning the "horny" part of its name—and increasing his nitric oxide production. Epimedium can also boost his libido by supporting his adrenal glands, and may have male hormone–like effects.

From a Chinese medicine perspective, epimedium is a very yang herb, recommended if a man needs to build his yang energy, so it may be best reserved for specific sexual-health issues. (Later in this chapter, we'll explore its use for treating erectile dysfunction.) Taking epimedium as a single herb may be beneficial in some cases, but could overstimulate a man's libido and eventually exhaust his energy; it's typically found in herbal formulas for increasing sexual vitality and overall health. If taken as a single herb, the recommended dose for men is 300 mg, standardized to contain at least 20 percent icariin, up to three times daily. A man should refrain from using epimedium if he has an overactive sex drive, high fever, insomnia, anxiety, or low blood pressure, or if he's on blood-thinning medications.

— *Tribulus terrestris.* An herb that grows in Africa and India, *Tribulus terrestris* has long been used by native peoples for its therapeutic effects on male libido. Modern research shows that its active compound, protodioscin, can act as a precursor to the hormones testosterone and DHEA. Bulgarian researchers demonstrated that the herb could increase levels of these hormones in men, although more research is needed to confirm this. Because it can increase nitric oxide, *Tribulus terrestris* has been found effective for treating erectile dysfunction. Research also supports its use for enhancing sperm quality and improving male fertility. The recommended daily dose for men is 85 to 250 mg with food. Look for products containing 45 percent protodioscin.

— **Ginkgo biloba.** Extracts from the seeds and the leaves of the ginkgo biloba tree, used in Asia since ancient times for aphrodisiac and healing purposes, can enhance a man's libido by increasing his nitric oxide level. As you discovered in Chapter 5, ginkgo biloba may also provide antioxidant benefits and a wide range of other potential health gains, including thinning the blood, strengthening blood-vessel walls, promoting circulation, and improving memory in older people.

The recommended dose for men is 40 mg three times daily, as a standardized extract of 24 percent ginkgo flavonglycosides. Side effects are unusual, but some people report minor headaches or stomachaches. Ginkgo biloba is well suited to most men, but shouldn't be taken by anyone on blood-thinning medications.

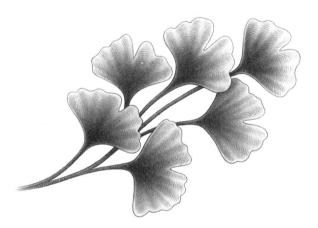

The characteristically crenellated leaves of the ginkgo biloba tree.

— **Maca.** The root of the maca plant has a lengthy history of use in Peru for increasing male sexual potency and endurance. Ample research supports its beneficial effects on a man's libido, sexual desire, fertility, and spermatogenesis. One study, published in *Andrologia* in 2002, found that maca improved sexual desire in men who took 1,500 to 3,000 mg for three months. Another study, published in the *Asian Journal of Andrology* in 2001, found that men who took maca for four months had improved sperm count, seminal-fluid volume, and sperm mobility. Research shows maca increases male potency without affecting production of testosterone and other hormones, and also helps relieve stress, support the adrenal glands, and reduce stress-hormone levels. The recommended dose for men is 2,000 mg twice daily. Researchers haven't reported any side effects from using it. (See Appendix C for supplier information.)

— **Yohimbine.** As you saw in Chapter 5, yohimbine is an aphrodisiac that works by stimulating blood flow and nerve impulses to the genitals. It is also a useful treatment for sexual dysfunction caused by some antidepressant drugs. Yohimbine is effective for both women and men, but can be especially potent for men. Research shows that it has promise for treating male impotence, and it's the only herb approved by the FDA for treating erectile dysfunction.

Yohimbine isn't safe for everyone, and needs to be taken within careful guidelines because of its potential toxicity. Anyone considering taking it should refer to its cautions and recommendations in Chapter 5. It shouldn't be taken along with some drugs or by men with certain health conditions, including prostate-gland problems such as benign prostatic hyperplasia. If taken in excess, or along with some foods and dietary items, it could have serious side effects. Before taking yohimbine (either in over-the-counter products or as the prescription drug yohimbine hydrochloride), it's best to see a doctor trained in its use. If a man is a candidate to use yohimbine hydrochloride, the dose typically prescribed for issues of sexual performance and erectile dysfunction is 5.4 mg three times daily.

— **Hot Plants for Him.** Hot Plants for Him, an over-the-counter herbal aphrodisiac formula, contains maca, yohimbe-bark extract, rhodiola, epimedium, Panax ginseng (Chinese ginseng), and tongkat ali. Most of these ingredients are aimed at building a man's libido by supporting his adrenal glands, increasing nitric oxide, and promoting neurotransmitters like serotonin. According to the company that makes it, the amount of yohimbine in the product is 4 percent, which would equal 4 mg of active constituent of yohimbine per pill. The label provides warnings, but extra care should be taken to avoid using more than the recommended dose of two pills daily. In excess, it could cause adverse effects, especially if taken with wine, cheese, or liver. Any man using this product should heed Chapter 5's cautions for taking yohimbine. (See Appendix C for supplier information.)

— **Male Libido.** Another over-the-counter herbal product, Male Libido contains a blend of epimedium, fo-ti, maca, sarsaparilla, saw palmetto, *Tribulus terrestris,* wild oats, and yohimbine. Again, a man using this product should bear in mind the precautions for taking yohimbine outlined in Chapter 5. (For supplier information, see Appendix C.)

Just Say *Yes* to NO

As touched upon in an earlier chapter, nitric oxide (NO) can enhance your sexual response because it dilates blood vessels that supply your vagina and vulva. NO plays a similar role in a man's sexual response. It's important for generating and maintaining erections because it dilates the blood vessels of his penis, promoting increased penile blood flow and sensitivity. A urine test can evaluate a man's NO production, and if he has erectile dysfunction, may help determine whether it's due to low NO synthesis in his penis. Known as a Urine NOx Test, it's available from Meridian Valley Lab. (See Appendix C.)

Other Male Aphrodisiacs and Enhancers: Supplements and Foods

Along with the nutritional supplements and dietary choices you explored in Chapter 2, which have the cumulative effect of creating a solid "platform" for a man's overall sexual health, certain supplements and foods can give his sexuality an added boost. First, let's look at some important sex-enhancing vitamins, minerals, and other supplements he can use:

215

— **Zinc.** Research shows that zinc, a key mineral for male sexual health and performance, promotes healthy testosterone levels, sperm count, and fertility, and that zinc deficiency can compromise male hormonal health. Zinc also supports a man's prostate gland, and is essential to many other functions in his body. The recommended dose is 25 to 50 mg daily.

— **Vitamin B$_6$ and magnesium.** These two nutrients help a man's body use zinc to support testosterone production. The recommended daily doses are 50 mg of B$_6$ and 500 mg of magnesium. (Note: Excessive magnesium may cause diarrhea in some people.)

— **L-arginine.** An essential amino acid, L-arginine can enhance a man's sexuality by increasing nitric oxide. Recommended doses are typically between 2,000 and 6,000 mg daily. A man should avoid taking L-arginine if he has low blood pressure, a gastric ulcer, liver disease, kidney disease, or genital herpes.

— **Vitamin E.** By helping to protect sperm from oxidative stress, vitamin E promotes male fertility. It also supports cardiovascular health and thins a man's blood, which helps prevent clogged blood vessels, including those that supply his penis and facilitate erections. The recommended dose is 400 IU daily.

— **DHEA.** DHEA, a precursor to testosterone (which means that it converts to testosterone in a man's body), can enhance male libido and help maintain erections. It's naturally produced in a man's body—much of it comes from his adrenal glands, although it's also made in his brain—and released into his bloodstream during orgasm. Taken in supplement form, DHEA can slightly raise testosterone levels in some men, and may increase feelings of well-being, boost energy, support memory functions, and help prevent heart disease. A laboratory test is needed to determine if a man's DHEA level is low. If so, recommended doses are typically between 25 and 50 mg daily.

— **Nettle root.** Research shows that nettle root can increase the amount of free testosterone a man has in circulation and help with an enlarged prostate gland by arresting prostate-cell growth. It can also positively affect the testosterone-to-estrogen ratio in the prostate gland and help with issues pertaining to *BPH,* an enlargement of the prostate gland that is a common condition we'll explore later in this chapter. The recommended dose is 300 mg daily.

— **Omega-3 fats.** Omega-3 fats convert into hormone-like substances called *prostaglandins* that are stored in high concentrations in a man's prostate gland, where they help decrease inflammation and prevent prostate-cell growth. Flax and fish oils are two of the best sources of omega-3 fats; the recommended daily dose for flax oil is one tablespoon containing 6,200 mg of omega-3 fats, and for fish oil an amount containing at least 500 mg of EPA and 300 mg of DHA.

— **Saw palmetto.** Studies show that extracts of saw-palmetto berries can promote a man's prostate-gland health and help reduce symptoms of BPH. While this may not seem to directly enhance his sexuality, by preventing common prostate issues, it can make an enormous difference in his ability to enjoy sex. The recommended daily dose is 320 mg of a standardized extract of saw palmetto.

In addition to these supplements, a few foods warrant special mention for their ability to provide an extra dose of male sexual-health enhancement. Some of the following appear elsewhere in this book due to their beneficial effects on female libido. Along with many of the same benefits you stand to reap from consuming them, they can give your partner added gains that apply uniquely to men's sexual-health issues.

— **Oysters.** Not only are oysters among the best natural sources of zinc, but they're also a good source of omega-3 fats and vitamins.

— **Pumpkin seeds.** As one of Chapter 2's super-libido foods, pumpkin seeds boost immunity, decrease cholesterol, promote bone strength, and may have anti-inflammatory effects. They offer additional benefits for a man's prostate gland: a study in the *British Journal of Urology* found that *curbicin,* a compound in pumpkin seeds, improves symptoms associated with BPH. And pumpkin seeds are also high in zinc, as well as prostate-friendly omega-3 fats.

The Aphrodisiac Potential of Pumpkin Pie:
Hiding in Plain Scent

Your sense of smell is intimately connected with your experience of sex; people who lose their sense of smell may have reduced sexual perceptiveness. Even though pumpkin seeds are good for your partner's sexual health, you might never guess that a smell associated with pumpkins can stimulate his sexual response. But when it comes to the olfactory sense, research suggests that pumpkins are indeed at it again. At Chicago's Smell and Taste Treatment Research Foundation, neurologist Alan Hirsch tested the effects of a wide variety of scents on sexual response in men, measured by blood flow to the penis. The test sample was relatively small, but the results were a big surprise. Of all scents tested, the greatest reaction was to that of pumpkin pie, which (along with lavender) elicited an increase in penile blood flow up to 40 percent. So next time you want to get your partner in the mood, consider whipping up a pumpkin pie for dessert. Maybe that old wives' tale should be amended: the way to a man's heart is through his stomach . . . *and nose.*

— **Oatmeal.** Oats are high in zinc, and they contain *beta-glucan,* a type of fiber that can help lower cholesterol, thereby supporting a man's sexual health by reducing his heart-disease risk. (Heart disease, which clogs blood vessels to the penis, can be a factor in impotence.)

— **Pomegranate juice.** Although pomegranates may not have specific aphrodisiac effects, they offer numerous advantages for male sexual health. They're high in antioxidants and other compounds that make them particularly beneficial for the prostate gland, and they may help prevent prostate cancer. Research published by the *Journal of Medicinal Food* shows that pomegranate-derived compounds have antitumor activity in the prostate, and a UCLA study of men with recurrent prostate cancer found that eight ounces of pomegranate juice consumed daily significantly reduced prostate-cancer growth, increased the death of cancer cells, and reduced their proliferation.

Pomegranate juice can also increase circulation, which (as you'll see in the pages ahead) may help improve male erectile response. Other benefits include reduced blood pressure and improved cardiovascular health (with the potential to reverse heart disease). Pomegranate juice gives a man an enjoyable, convenient way to consume the fruit's beneficial ingredients in a readily absorbable form.

Soy and Conception

If you and your partner are trying to conceive, he may want to avoid eating lots of soy. A study published in the journal *Human Reproduction* in 2009 found that a high intake of soy foods is associated with lower sperm concentrations, although it didn't affect sperm-cell quality or semen volume. According to the study, decreases in sperm concentration were especially pronounced in obese men who ate high-soy diets.

Rekindling Passion by Overcoming Erectile Dysfunction

You may not often find informative articles about natural solutions to erectile dysfunction (ED) in popular health magazines, but it's one of the more prevalent conditions in the United States, estimated to affect 17 percent of men in their 60s and close to half over 75. A man who has ED, once more widely referred to as *impotence,* is either unable to have an erection or unable to maintain one sufficient for satisfactory sex. He may also have reduced libido, although not necessarily. To be diagnosed as having ED, a man has to experience a frequent or consistent inability to have or maintain erections. ED is usually considered severe if a man is rarely able to have erections, and mild if he can sometimes have them. (If your partner is only occasionally unable to achieve or maintain an erection, it doesn't mean he has ED.)

In addition to the obvious problems it can create for a man's sex life, ED can also affect his quality of life and self-esteem. Many men feel they're expected to be always "up" for sex, literally. If a man finds himself unable to rise to the occasion, so to speak, it can have profound implications for his sense of self. If your partner has ED, or any episode where he's unable to have or maintain an erection, it's important to use sensitivity and avoid any emotional trauma or shame around sexual-performance issues.

ED can have many causes and contributing factors: damaged nerves that supply the penis, heart disease (such as hardening of the arteries) that reduces blood flow to the penis, the use of common prescription medications (including antidepressants, appetite suppressants, and high-blood-pressure drugs), obesity, poor diet, hypertension, poor nitric oxide production, hormone imbalances (including low testosterone, which we'll address later in this chapter), midlife hormone changes, unrelenting stress, enervating illnesses, and psychological issues. A man is at greater risk for ED if he smokes; uses alcohol to excess; or has pelvic surgery, diabetes, radiation therapy, nerve disorders, or strokes. And a recent study in the *International Journal of Men's Health* found that circumcised men are more than four times more likely to experience ED than intact men.

There are many solutions to ED, and plenty of reasons for a man with ED to be optimistic about overcoming it. Both Western natural medicine and Chinese medicine, as you'll discover, can provide effective alternatives for addressing many of the underlying causes. (Some, such as damaged nerves to the penis, may require special medical attention; a man who has ED should have a doctor do a checkup to determine the cause and rule out serious conditions.)

Prescription drugs like Viagra, Cialis, and Levitra have been aggressively marketed for men with ED, but they're hardly natural. (See sidebar.) A man who treats ED with natural methods is apt to find them vastly preferable to drugs because he won't be dependent on taking a pill prior to sex. Rather than feeling like a man who has ED and needs oral medication as a temporary fix, he'll feel that his sexual function is more or less back to normal.

Drugs like Viagra certainly aren't panaceas for ED. For some men, their effects diminish over time, or they never succeed to begin with. If a man's ED is caused by psychological factors (an estimated 20 percent of cases fit this category), it often involves complex emotional and relationship issues that no drug can unravel, and requires more than a chemical approach. In such situations, drugs like Viagra can be futile attempts to remove symptoms without resolving underlying problems, which need psychological solutions. And it's no small irony that many cases of ED are caused by side effects of prescription drugs, yet met with more of the same. If side effects of one drug are "treated" by another with new side effects, at what point will the cycle end?

The Side Effects of Pharma-Sex

The potential side effects of drugs like Viagra can be frightening. They shouldn't be used by men who take nitrate drugs commonly prescribed for angina—the combination could cause potentially life-threatening drops in blood pressure—and some men with serious kidney or liver problems should be closely monitored for possible dangerous side effects.

You've probably seen the commercials for Viagra with a voice-over reciting a litany of warnings and side effects so lengthy that it seems to take up most of the ad time. The possible side effects mentioned on the manufacturer's website include headaches, stomachaches, facial flushing, sensitivity to light, dizziness, ringing in the ears, hearing loss, blurred vision and cyanopsia (seeing everything with a bluish tint), potentially dangerous abnormal heart rhythms, inability to lose an erection (considered a medical emergency), heart attacks, strokes, and death. Other sources list additional side effects that include chest pain, fainting, nosebleeds, rashes, shortness of breath, high blood pressure, low blood pressure, heart palpitations, cerebrovascular hemorrhage (bleeding into the brain's tissue), and transient ischemic attack (sudden temporary brain-function loss). Studies also link Viagra with loss of vision; in 2005, after blindness was reported by some men taking Viagra and similar drugs, the FDA requested that "vision loss" be added to the lists of possible side effects.

The consequences of taking Viagra and similar pharmaceutical ED treatments aren't always limited to their required warnings. If a long-established couple has grown accustomed to a certain frequency of sexual intimacy and a drug like Viagra is suddenly added to the mix, it can throw their relationship off balance. Although these drugs may seem like the answer for some couples, not every woman enjoys her partner's newfound drug-induced sexual interest; some complain that they can't, or don't want to, keep up with it. And a drug that unnaturally fuels sex can create other unexpected health problems, including increased rates of sexually transmitted infections among certain age-groups. (See Appendix G.)

You might wonder why ED should be treated at all, if men naturally experience hormonal changes and lower sexual function during some phases of their lives. Why not accept that ED is more common in older men, and let nature run its course? The answer is that many cases of ED aren't part of the natural aging process and are totally preventable. A man's sexuality may be different from the way it once was, but he doesn't necessarily have to settle for lower sexual function.

If a man learns he has ED because of heart disease, smoking, alcoholism, or the use of appetite-suppressant drugs, the bad news comes with a bright silver lining: since his condition is caused partly or entirely by unhealthy habits, lifestyle changes can be essential to reversing it. (His diagnosis may even give him the opportunity to take steps that save his life; ED is sometimes the first sign of a problem that, if left untreated, could eventually lead to heart attacks or strokes.) One or more changes in his habits and routines, applied consistently over time, may be all that's required to overcome ED. Let's look at the key lifestyle adjustments he might need to make and some tips that may help alleviate his condition:

— **Choose a heart-healthy, libido-boosting lifestyle.** First and foremost, healthy lifestyle choices mean eating right and getting enough exercise. A man with lifestyle-induced ED should be especially vigilant about adhering to every part of the Great Sex Lifestyle in Chapter 2. Pomegranate juice, which can increase blood flow, may particularly benefit men with ED resulting from clogged blood vessels. A 2005 study in the *Journal of Urology* found that pomegranate juice (in conjunction with other high-antioxidant drinks) helped improve erectile response.

— **Give up smoking and alcohol.** A man can treat ED not only with what he consumes and does, but also what he *doesn't* consume and do. If he's a smoker, he can wear a nicotine patch, use nicotine gum, or get acupuncture to help him quit. If he drinks alcohol, he can reduce his consumption, and avoid social functions involving heavy alcohol use. If he drinks excessively, he can get professional help, join a support group, or do whatever it takes to detoxify his body—and let ED be a "sobering" experience. Alcohol may be a factor in ED even if a man doesn't consider himself an alcoholic.

— **Relax!** A man who has ED is often a driven, goal-oriented individual who overstresses his system. The only thing he may not be driven to achieve is the state of relaxation necessary to regenerate his health and libido. When faced with ED, he may become even more focused on achievement elsewhere in his life and even less able to relax and relieve stress. It may be crucial for him to break out of this negative feedback loop and rediscover the value of taking time off for activities that aren't achievement related. He may benefit from stress-management courses or learning to meditate, but most of all he needs to forget about his worldly concerns, relax, and completely let go of the "fight" for a few hours every now and then. He may be surprised by how much this can affect his ability to enjoy sex again; some men are amazed to discover the degree to which, at times, leisure is the measure of pleasure.

— **Have more fun.** Some men with lifestyle-induced ED have lost sight of the simple joys of play and gleefulness. They may be out of touch with the hidden connections between sexuality and whimsicality, sensuality and impracticality, the erotic and the quixotic. Often men in this category need to remember how to discover the important links between fully enjoying life and being sexually functional—how to find the "fun" in functional.

— **Avoid vicious cycling.** If a man with ED is a cyclist or mountain biker, he may need to use bike seats that protect his lower pelvis and prevent pressure on the area between his scrotum and anus. Prolonged pressure on this area can compress blood vessels that supply the penis and lead to penile numbness and ED. (Some research suggests that constant seat vibration from extended motorcycle riding could also damage pelvic nerves.) A man who's in great shape from cycling may tend to exacerbate penile numbness and ED by mistakenly assuming that increasing, rather than decreasing, his workouts will relieve his symptoms.

— **Consider foreskin restoration.** In some cases of ED, penile sensitivity may be a contributing factor. According to a recent report in *Men's Health News,* circumcision severs the penile nerves responsible for most of a man's sexual sensory input, resulting in a reduction in penile sensitivity by as much as 75 percent. If your partner was circumcised, foreskin-restoration techniques, which we'll explore in the pages ahead, may help resolve ED by enhancing the sensitivity of his penis.

✼✼✼

While many men completely reverse ED with lifestyle changes, not all do. Men who have ED due to diabetes, for example, may not experience full recovery—but by making the right lifestyle choices, they can help manage both their ED and their diabetes. Similarly, some men who have ED as a result of being on drugs such as antidepressants or blood-pressure medications may find that healthy lifestyle changes don't reverse the condition, but make a difference in their ED as well as every other aspect of their lives. More important, men taking drugs that cause ED should, whenever possible, use natural medicines instead. A study issued online in 2011 by the *British Journal of Urology International* reported that the more prescription drugs a man takes, the greater his chances of having ED.

Along with lifestyle changes, a number of herbs and nutritional supplements can be helpful to any man with ED. Some work by boosting nitric oxide (which can be a factor in ED) or by exerting other beneficial effects. And unlike Viagra and similar drugs, they're not known to have any potentially life-threatening side effects when used properly.

As you've seen, the herbal aphrodisiac *Tribulus terrestris* is effective for men with ED because of its ability to increase nitric oxide; one study found it useful for treating ED in men with diabetes. (See recommendations for dosage and use earlier in this chapter.) And L-arginine, which we've explored for general male sexuality enhancement, can also help men with ED. A study reported in the *Journal of Sex & Marital Therapy* found that L-arginine combined with pycnogenol (a flavonoid derived from pine bark that can also affect a man's nitric oxide level) significantly improved ability to have and maintain erections in 92.5 percent of participants with ED. The recommended daily doses for treating ED, based on the study, are 1.7 grams of L-arginine and 80 mg of pycnogenol. (See earlier recommendations for taking L-arginine.)

In addition to *Tribulus terrestris,* L-arginine, and pycnogenol, the following are recommended for a man with ED. They've been found to be generally safe to use, and can be taken simultaneously.

— **L-citrulline.** An amino acid that increases nitric oxide synthesis, L-citrulline promotes healthy erections. Some researchers hypothesize that L-citrulline, which converts into L-arginine in a man's body, may be more effective than L-arginine because of the way the body metabolizes it. If L-arginine doesn't sufficiently improve a man's erections to allow him fulfilling sex, he may benefit from taking the recommended daily dose of 500 mg of L-citrulline. The only potential side effect is decreased blood pressure.

— **Acetyl-l-carnitine and propionyl L-carnitine.** Acetyl-l-carnitine and propionyl L-*carnitine* supplements are recommended for treating ED by Dr. Jonathan Wright, who pioneered the use of bioidentical testosterone for men. He suggests that men use 2,000 mg of each daily, instead of drugs like Viagra. Interestingly, studies published in the journal *Urology* have shown that when men whose prostate glands are removed (which can lead to ED) take these supplements along with Viagra, the drug becomes more effective. According to Dr. Wright, both supplements also increase cognitive and muscle function.

Understanding Andropause

Just as your sexuality changes as you travel through the seasons of your life, with your hormonal shifts and evolving emotional needs, a man goes through hormonal changes of his own. His midlife transition is less obvious than yours because there's no outward physical manifestation, like the cessation of menstrual cycles, but it deeply impacts some men nonetheless. During *andropause*, or male menopause, which typically begins between the ages of 45 and 55 (preceded by gradual hormonal changes that we call *periandropause*), there are shifts in a man's levels of testosterone, adrenal hormones, estrogen, and progesterone. These changes present few problems for some men, but great challenges for others. Over a period of several years, a happy, outgoing man may slowly become a less satisfied person who has difficulty concentrating and sleeping, gains weight easily, frequently feels exhausted, no longer seems to care about what once mattered to him, goes through a midlife crisis, has a diminished sex drive, or experiences ED.

It's important to remember that the changes a man experiences during andropause are a normal part of life; like menopause, andropause is natural, and not an illness. The changes may require acceptance and adaptation, but it's very possible for men to learn to be content with their new, physiologically altered postandropausal selves.

Together, andropause and menopause can test a relationship. With your two sexual energies in flux, the balance between you can shift in unforeseeable ways. Some long-term couples have settled into familiar patterns of sexual expression, only to find themselves going through physiological and emotional transitions that deeply affect their relationship. If both partners experience life-altering changes at the same time, they may feel that maintaining their sexual intimacy is like aiming at a moving target. But the fact that men and women go through these transitions at corresponding stages of their lives can also give them new opportunities to grow *together* rather than apart. It allows them to evolve together through parallel changes, to some extent mirroring each other, and their shared experiences can deepen and strengthen their partnership as they move through time.

Solutions to ED from Chinese Medicine

When it comes to men's sexual-health issues, Chinese medicine has a lot to say. ED is seen as the result of an underlying imbalance in a man's chi—especially a deficiency of his yang energy. If he takes drugs like Viagra to maintain erections, the underlying imbalance remains; having drug-assisted sex without addressing it only further imbalances his chi and depletes his yang energy, causing worse ED, and lower overall health, in the long run. By balancing his chi and boosting his yang energy, however, he can often get to the root of the problem.

In the West, we often think about a man's erection in a binary sense: either he has one or he doesn't. This either-or mentality is quite at odds with the way Chinese medicine approaches men's sexual health and ED. The *quality* of erections is seen as an essential factor in determining a man's sexual health. Firm, "hot" erections are a strong indicator that his chi and yang energy are abundant and well nourished; semi-flaccid erections are a sign that they're deficient. (Another important factor in evaluating a man's sexual health is the way he feels after orgasm. If he feels completely exhausted and falls asleep, it means he's chi-deficient.)

As you've discovered, Chinese medicine teaches that many lifestyle choices can balance chi and support yang energy. Along with the steps outlined previously in this book for a sex-supportive lifestyle, acupressure can help a man with ED address its underlying causes. To use acupressure to support yang energy and treat

ED, you or your partner can press firmly for a few minutes, once or twice daily, on these points on his body: Kidney 27, Kidney 1, Kidney 7, and San Jiao 4. (To locate these points, see Appendix A.)

In addition, certain Chinese herbs can be effective for treating ED, either by boosting a man's yang energy or because of their other beneficial effects. Let's look at the most important options a man can try. (In the preceding pages you've explored some of these herbs for general male sex enhancement; here we examine them specifically for their ED-alleviating effects.) A man with ED may need to take these herbs for three to six months to experience many of their benefits.

— **Chinese ginseng.** Research shows Chinese ginseng can be highly beneficial for men with ED. A study published in the *Journal of Urology* in 2002, which found significant reductions of ED symptoms over a 16-week course of treatment, concluded that the herb is an effective ED treatment. Another study, published in *Clinical Autonomic Research* in 2001, reported that Chinese ginseng increases nitric oxide production in the delicate blood vessels lining the corpus cavernosum, the spongy erectile tissue of the penis (dilation of this tissue with blood is necessary for erection), and also positively affects other naturally occurring compounds in the body that may allow for improved penile blood flow. Chinese ginseng provides these benefits without causing changes in blood levels of testosterone. (See dosage and use recommendations earlier in this chapter.)

— **Lu Rong.** Although often referred to as an herb, Lu Rong is derived from deer antlers. Chinese physicians have used Lu Rong for thousands of years, usually combined with other ingredients in herbal formulas, to build yang energy, fortify libido, increase longevity, and strengthen the entire body. In recent times, it has been used by athletes to improve performance, strength, and muscle mass. It also has immune-enhancing functions, promotes sound sleep, and boosts endurance. Research shows it's high in mucopolysaccharides, which can help regenerate tissue, and rich in IGF, a substance similar to growth hormone that helps the body recuperate more quickly from exercise. One formula containing Lu Rong, a product known as Antler 8, is used to treat ED, as well as lowered immunity and arthritis. The recommended dose is two pills three times daily; see Appendix C for supplier information. (Note: Animals aren't harmed in the collection of Lu Rong.)

— **Epimedium.** As mentioned earlier in this chapter, the active constituent of this yang-building herb, found in many Chinese herbal formulas used to treat ED, is icariin. Not only can icariin help a man with ED by stimulating nerves to his genitals and increasing nitric oxide, but it has other anti-ED benefits as well. In 2003, the *Asian Journal of Andrology* published research showing that icariin positively influences blood flow to the penis and effectively treats ED through its effects on an enzyme that allows for smooth muscle relaxation of the corpus cavernosum— interestingly, the same way Viagra works. (See recommendations for epimedium's dosage and use earlier in this chapter.)

— **Ginkgo biloba.** For a man with ED as a side effect of taking antidepressant drugs, ginkgo biloba can be especially beneficial. A study reported in *Alternative Medicine Review* found it 76 percent effective in alleviating symptoms associated with every phase of the sexual-response cycle, including symptoms of ED, in men with antidepressant-induced sexual dysfunction. Another study, published in the *Journal of Sex & Martial Therapy,* supported these results. The recommended daily dose for treating ED is 200 mg, as a standardized extract of 24 percent ginkgo flavonglycosides. (See usage guidelines described previously in this chapter.)

— **Herbal formulas.** Some Chinese formulas include various combinations of Chinese ginseng, Lu Rong, or epimedium, making them valuable for treating ED. One formula, called Man's Treasure (also known as *Nan Bao Pian*)—which contains Chinese ginseng, epimedium, and other nourishing herbs—is recommended for treating male impotence and infertility, as well as fatigue and premature aging. The recommended dose is two pills three times daily. Another formula, Male Function, includes Chinese ginseng, Lu Rong, epimedium, and other herbs that stimulate chi and increase circulation. The recommended dose is four capsules three times daily. (Note: Either of these formulas, if taken by a man who doesn't have ED, could cause overstimulation, which can ultimately lead to depleted chi and low libido.) For resources for Chinese herbal formulas, see Appendix C.

In this chapter, you haven't yet explored one of the other important issues that can cause or contribute to ED—a low testosterone level. For some men, ED can be a symptom of low testosterone. If ED is associated with low libido or occurs around midlife, low testosterone is especially likely to be a factor. Low testosterone is a separate challenge unto itself, and so vital to a man's sexual health that it deserves special attention; we'll devote the next section to a detailed exploration. If a man's ED is due to a low testosterone level, he can treat this cause with methods mapped out in the following pages.

Resolving Low Testosterone: The Joys of Renewed Libido

Men and testosterone are inextricably linked. This hormone is an integral part of what you love about your partner; it shapes his masculine nature, musculature, deeper voice, and attraction to you. You want him to have testosterone, but just the right amount. Too much, or too little, can throw off the natural balance, affect both of your sex lives, and create hormonal havoc. The good news is that there's a lot he can do to maintain his healthy testosterone level, and a lot you can do to support him.

You have testosterone in your body, too, and as you saw earlier in this book, it plays an important role in your sexual health. Testosterone affects both males and females, and before puberty boys and girls have about the same levels in their blood. At puberty, testosterone increases in both sexes, but it surges in boys.

In a man's body, testosterone is made primarily by the testicles. It travels through the bloodstream, acts on many organs and tissues, and provides numerous health benefits. Studies show that men with normal or high testosterone levels are more likely to have healthy blood vessels, and may live longer than those with low testosterone levels. Low testosterone is associated with obesity, diabetes, and increased risks for cardiovascular disease and heart attacks.

Testosterone is essential for the functions of your partner's sex organs, including his penis, testicles, prostate gland, and seminal vesicles. His penis contains testosterone receptors that release chemical signals to help with erections, and testosterone is important for his sperm production, and involved in ejaculation. Testosterone also affects his entire body by increasing the size and strength of his muscle cells, helping reduce his body fat, and playing an important role in maintaining his long-term bone strength.

Your partner's brain also has testosterone receptors, and they affect how he thinks—including his sexual thoughts about you. Testosterone is critical to the complex tapestry of biological and psychological factors we call "desire." If your partner has low testosterone, it may be influencing your relationship in more ways than you would expect, because it can affect his moods, motivation, and attitude toward life. In some cases, the symptoms can be enormously challenging; remember that he needs your support and compassion. In the pages ahead we'll explore the key issues around low testosterone, what you need to know if your partner has the condition, and what can be done to resolve it.

Could His Testosterone Level Be Affecting Your Relationship?

Low testosterone—the reduction in the amount of testosterone in a man's bloodstream to a subnormal level—is more common than many people realize. It can occur at any age, but it's most often caused by the natural decline in testosterone in a man's body, beginning in his mid-30s, by about one percent a year. An estimated 10 percent of 40-year-olds, 20 percent of 50-year-olds, and 30 percent of 60-year-olds have low testosterone, although a lesser number may have the symptoms. Decreases in testosterone are most likely to be caused by the hormonal shifts of andropause, when a man's testosterone-to-estrogen ratio can change dramatically, from as high as 50 to 1 to as low as 8 to 1.

If your partner has low testosterone, it can impact many aspects of your sex life and your relationship. The symptom he's most likely to notice is decreased sex drive; he doesn't desire sexual intimacy as often or passionately as he once did, or feels no interest whatsoever. He may have an absence of sexual responsiveness or "spark," even in situations he formerly found arousing. The decline can be so gradual that it goes unnoticed. It can be difficult to compare the memory of a man's sex drive of many years ago with what it is today, and he may have forgotten what it's like to have normal libido.

You may also notice that your partner seems fatigued and irritable more often than he used to. He may have less overall vitality and energy, lack motivation and enthusiasm, laugh less frequently, seem to enjoy life less, or describe himself as feeling "old." These mood changes can be pervasive, last for extended periods of time, and affect all of your conversations and experiences with him.

If your partner's low testosterone leads to symptoms of ED, he may need to concentrate to maintain an erection, and sex may seem to him like it's all "work"—or it may not work at all. If he's able to have an orgasm, it may be diminished in intensity. Some men with unusually low levels of testosterone also have low sperm counts or decreased quantities of semen.

Men with low testosterone often experience loss of muscle and strength. Your partner may notice that his muscles don't respond to exercise the way they once did, even though he works out as much as before, or that it takes longer for his body to recover after workouts. In addition, even if he hasn't changed his eating habits, he may accumulate extra body fat, especially around the waist, that can't be shed regardless of how conscientiously he exercises.

There's no single symptom that definitively and necessarily means your partner has low testosterone; symptoms can vary widely from one man to another. Some men with low testosterone have only one symptom, while others have many. Some may not have the primary symptom, low sex drive, but still have low testosterone. If your partner seems to have one or more symptoms, it's important to remember that they can all have causes unrelated to testosterone levels, such as normal aging, other health conditions, stress, depression, or side effects of prescription drugs. For instance, if a man is on the type of antidepressants known as selective serotonin reuptake inhibitors (for example, Prozac), the side effects can include lowered sex drive and difficulty reaching orgasm.

Low testosterone is treatable and potentially reversible, but according to the FDA only about 5 percent of American men with the condition receive treatment. Despite its prevalence, the conventional medical establishment has been slow to offer clear guidelines for diagnosis and treatment. Millions of men with the

231

symptoms don't have dependable sources of information, and many physicians, uncertain about how to accurately determine if men have low testosterone, may dismiss or misdiagnose their complaints. In addition, some physicians don't feel comfortable treating a decline in testosterone because it's seen as a normal part of aging. This is odd, because we take elaborate steps to compensate for normal aspects of aging in many other ways—for instance, with our vision, teeth, hearing, hearts, and joints—and do whatever we can to improve the quality of our lives in all these areas. Yet if low testosterone significantly reduces a person's quality of life, many doctors seem unconcerned.

Fortunately, times are changing. There's growing awareness of the importance of low testosterone, and more willingness on the part of some doctors to diagnose and treat it when appropriate.

Late Sex, Naturally: Pleasure and Older Couples

Studies show that the primary reasons older couples stop being sexually active are poor health and a tendency to simply lose interest in sex. Low testosterone and reduced sex drive may often be a factor. Who are "older" couples? By some definitions you qualify if you're over 60, but as the saying goes, you're only as old as you feel. If you consistently follow the lifestyle recommendations earlier in this book, you could vastly increase your likelihood of being sexually active in your 60s; your overall health can be the single most important factor in your ability to keep the *sex* in sexagenarian.

If you're 70 or older, the pleasures and health benefits of sex can still be yours. Research shows that about seven out of ten couples enjoy sex in their 70s, and some well into their 80s. Again, being especially vigilant about your health can make all the difference; the higher your age, the more your cumulative lifestyle choices may determine your potential to enjoy being sexually active. In your golden years, great health is invaluable, and wise choices can yield particularly rich rewards for your ability to savor the treasure of pleasure.

The Potential Benefits of Treating Low Testosterone for Both Your Partner and Yourself

For many men, increasing testosterone levels and alleviating symptoms of low testosterone completely changes their lives. If your partner has the condition, the right solution can transform *your* life as well. Just as the symptoms of low testosterone can permeate every aspect of your relationship, the benefits of treatment can affect each moment, activity, and conversation you share. Not every man shows dramatic improvements, and not every symptom is resolved—libido depends on many biological and psychological factors in addition to testosterone—but for many men it can restore the ability to have not only a satisfying sex life but a more fulfilling life in general. Let's look at the benefits your partner may experience from treatment if he has low testosterone:

— **Increased sex drive and sexual function.** When a man's testosterone level is restored to normal, he often experiences a rebirth of desire, more frequent interest in sex, and greater ability to become aroused. He may have a renewed sense that sex, after all, should be perennial, *not* sexennial (occurring every six years). And as previous pages have touched on, if he has ED, increased testosterone may partly or completely resolve it.

— **Mood enhancements.** Men who restore their testosterone levels often describe feeling more youthful, "masculine," mentally alert, creative, and alive; they tend to use adjectives like *energetic, vigorous, recharged,* and *rejuvenated.* Many report newfound sensations of well-being, overall self-confidence, and zest for life. Their partners often find them happier, more pleasant, and less irritable.

— **Greater lean muscle mass.** Many studies have found that increased testosterone improves overall muscle bulk. Not only does it enlarge each muscle cell, but it may also create more muscle by "recruiting" nearby cells to become muscle cells. Due to increased lean muscle mass, men who restore their testosterone levels may also experience increased overall body weight.

— **Increased muscle strength.** Research shows testosterone treatment can increase muscle strength, even without exercise. One study found a 17 percent increase without exercise, and a 27 percent increase with exercise. Men who restore their testosterone levels often experience measurable improvements in their workouts and reduced workout-recovery time.

— **Body-fat reduction.** At the same time that testosterone increases lean muscle mass, it reduces body fat—especially belly fat.

— **Improved bone density.** If a man has decreased bone density due to low testosterone, treatment with testosterone can gradually improve his bone density.

If your partner has low testosterone, improvements may begin to be noticed within the first few months of treatment and are likely to stay in effect for as long as his testosterone level remains restored. Men who seek testosterone treatment for a particular symptom, such as low libido or difficulty maintaining erections, often experience unexpected benefits in other areas of their lives.

How to Determine If a Man Has Low Testosterone

If your partner has one or more of the symptoms described above, and if there are no other obvious reasons for his symptoms, he can determine whether he has low testosterone by having a doctor order blood tests that measure his levels of total testosterone, free testosterone, and estrogen. Two other blood tests, a sex hormone binding globulin (SHBG) test and a prostate-specific antigen (PSA) test, are also helpful, especially if he's considering testosterone replacement treatment, which we'll explore in the pages ahead. Another test, not typically done by conventional physicians, is a comprehensive urine hormone test that measures testosterone and other hormones over a 24-hour period. This test provides much more information, including levels of testosterone, DHEA, progesterone, estrogen, and cortisol.

If these tests indicate a man has low testosterone, he's a candidate for treatment—perhaps testosterone replacement—to elevate his testosterone level. At this point, it's recommended that he have a doctor do additional tests to look for a possible explanation for his low testosterone: a luteinizing hormone test (to show if his pituitary gland is functioning correctly in regard to testosterone production) and a prolactin test (to rule out a rare pituitary gland tumor). If these tests come back showing normal results, he stands to gain from treatment methods as described in the following section.

Natural Solutions for Low Testosterone

If a man has one or more characteristic symptoms of low testosterone, and if blood and urine tests confirm low or borderline levels of either total or free testosterone, he may benefit from some form of treatment. In some cases, men with low testosterone don't need to increase their testosterone levels; some have no symptoms, and increasing their testosterone may have no clear benefits. But if a man wants to change his condition, there are many steps he can take and many options available.

As with so many health issues, it makes sense to begin with natural treatments—the most conservative, gentlest, and safest methods—before considering other measures. Conventional doctors, who are trained to prescribe pharmaceutical and synthetic products, may be biased against natural approaches, but a growing body of evidence shows that natural therapies can be effective for many men with low testosterone. All natural methods give a man the satisfaction of avoiding the risks of taking synthetic testosterone, and some allow him to restore his own testosterone level with do-it-yourself approaches.

Let's begin by exploring the gentlest of the natural treatments—the ways a man can enhance his testosterone production with lifestyle, diet, exercise, nutritional supplements, and herbs:

— **Lifestyle.** Along with the lifestyle tips you discovered earlier in this book, most of the lifestyle recommendations we've explored for treating ED can also benefit a man with low testosterone. From the Chinese medicine perspective, a balanced lifestyle is essential; a life of excess exhausts a man's chi, which can lead to premature aging and symptoms of decreased testosterone. Sleep is also important: a study published in 2011 in the *Journal of the American Medical Association* found that young men who slept fewer than five hours a night for eight consecutive nights averaged a 10 to 15 percent reduction in testosterone levels and experienced symptoms of low testosterone.

— **Diet.** Many people are unaware that a man's diet can either reduce or boost his testosterone level. If your partner joins you in following the diet recommended in Chapter 2, it will go a long way toward supporting his natural testosterone production by helping keep his body fat under control. This is a key issue in testosterone production; men with increased abdominal fat have higher levels of estrogen, which causes decreased testosterone.

— **Exercise.** Research shows regular exercise can be beneficial as a means of boosting a man's testosterone. It not only promotes testosterone production by helping prevent abdominal fat, but also mollifies cortisol, the testosterone-lowering stress hormone. Exercise is an effective natural, inexpensive way of increasing testosterone, and provides a wide range of other health gains.

Can Watching Sports Raise Your Partner's Testosterone Level?

Recent research may explain why your partner loves watching sports. If his team wins, according to a 2010 report in the journal *Psychoneuroendocrinology,* his testosterone level rises. So next time you think he's spending too much time glued to the sports channels, try reframing the issue: maybe he's not a couch potato after all, but a conscientious partner ardently working on improving your sex life by upping his testosterone level.

— **Supplements.** As you've seen, zinc is important for a man's testosterone level, vitamins B_6 and magnesium support testosterone production, and DHEA may raise testosterone levels in some men. (See recommendations for dosage and use described previously in this chapter.)

— **Herbal remedies.** In our exploration of the herbal aphrodisiacs tongkat ali and *Tribulus terrestris,* we pointed out their potential for increasing a man's testosterone level. (See dose and usage guidelines earlier in this chapter.) Suma can also be used, as recommended for aphrodisiac purposes in Chapter 5, to increase testosterone in men. And two Chinese herbal formulas you discovered in the preceding pages for treating ED, Man's Treasure and Male Function, may also help some men with low testosterone.

Natural Bioidentical Testosterone Treatment

If a man has tried natural lifestyle methods for at least three months but still experiences symptoms, and tests have confirmed low or borderline levels of total or free testosterone, he may want to pursue testosterone treatment. In the right circumstances, it can help him immeasurably. If he also has low libido or ED as a result of low testosterone, natural testosterone may not only boost his libido and treat ED but also improve his overall vitality. One patient's account of her partner's experience is typical: "He just didn't seem to have his mojo anymore; he was often tired and aloof about things he once loved. I never realized his moods were due to low testosterone. After tests showed his level was low and he starting natural testosterone, he said he never felt so good—and our once-passionate sex life returned."

Any man considering using testosterone needs to know the crucial distinction between natural testosterone and its synthetic counterpart. Natural testosterone is called "bioidentical" because it's composed of the same kind of molecules a man's own body produces over the course of his lifetime, as opposed to the chemically altered version found in synthetic testosterone products. Synthetic testosterone is neither natural nor bioidentical—testosterone expert Dr. Jonathan Wright says it doesn't qualify as a real hormone—and has a host of potential side effects, health risks, and safety issues that can be avoided by using natural testosterone. Natural testosterone is preferable to synthetic for the same reasons that natural bioidentical hormones are preferable for women: it's always better to use molecules as close as possible to nature and to the ones your body naturally makes.

Natural testosterone is safe and effective if used with the guidance of a qualified health-care professional who can help a man determine the right dose and monitor his treatment. A man who wants to take natural testosterone needs to find a doctor trained in natural hormone treatment. (A prescription is required.) Licensed naturopathic physicians are typically well versed on current natural methods; see Appendix B to find a qualified practitioner. To explore methods of taking testosterone, recommended doses, and follow-up testing, see Appendix I.

Further Considerations: Other Potential Benefits and Effects of Natural Testosterone Treatment

— **Heart-health advantages?** Some concerns have been raised that increasing testosterone might elevate risk of heart disease in men, but research indicates that many risk factors for cardiovascular disease, such as hypertension, cholesterol, obesity, and high blood sugar, may be greater in men with *low* testosterone. In *Maximize Your Vitality & Potency,* Dr. Jonathan Wright and Lane Lenard cite multiple studies showing that natural testosterone treatment significantly decreases total cholesterol and unfriendly LDL cholesterol. And higher testosterone levels seem to protect against atherosclerosis, while low levels may be a risk factor. There appears to be growing evidence that normal testosterone levels are beneficial for heart health.

— **Potential side effects.** Although natural testosterone is safer than synthetic testosterone, it's not without some of the potential side effects that synthetic testosterone has:

- First, for some men there may be overconversion of testosterone to its by-product dihydrotestosterone (DHT), which can cause increased head-hair loss. This potential effect can be prevented or mitigated by using saw palmetto, in the same dose recommended earlier in this chapter for general sexuality enhancement.

- Second, testosterone treatment may decrease a man's natural sperm production, although sperm count is typically restored within three to six months after discontinuing treatment. This may be an advantage for couples who don't want to conceive, but men with concerns about infertility, or who are being treated for it, shouldn't use testosterone.

- Third, some men experience acne during testosterone treatment, as a result of increased oil production in the skin; this typically decreases after several months of use.

- Finally, as described in Appendix I, some men may have skin irritation when using gels, creams, and patches.

— **Prostate issues.** It was once generally thought that testosterone treatment could increase a man's risk of prostate cancer by accelerating growth of prostate-cancer cells, but new evidence suggests that testosterone treatment is prostate-safe. As a 2004 article in the *New England Journal of Medicine* pointed out, "there appears to be no compelling evidence at present to suggest that men with higher testosterone levels are at greater risk of prostate cancer." Harvard professor Abraham Morgentaler, M.D., writes in *Testosterone for Life* that "although it has been widely believed for several decades that higher testosterone levels are associated with prostate cancer risks, it turns out there is no scientific evidence that this is true." Despite this, some doctors still cling to the belief that testosterone treatment is linked with prostate cancer.

There are growing concerns that prostate-cancer risk could be higher for men with *low* testosterone. Morgentaler goes on to say that "men are at increased risk for prostate cancer when they are older and their testosterone levels have declined. Men never develop prostate cancer when they are young and their testosterone levels are at their lifetime peak. New evidence suggests that low testosterone, rather than high testosterone, may be a risk for prostate cancer."

It has also long been assumed that testosterone treatment could pose concerns for men with a history of prostate cancer and put them at increased risk. Because of this, all testosterone treatment products bear an FDA-required warning that they're contraindicated in men with prior history of prostate cancer. Some studies in recent years, however, have indicated that testosterone treatment may be safer than once thought for men in this category. Today, some doctors may prescribe testosterone to men who have previously been treated for prostate cancer.

Along with the myth that testosterone treatment increases risk of prostate cancer, there has been a widespread belief that it could result in benign growth of the prostate gland (also known as *BPH*, which we'll look at in the pages ahead). But numerous studies have

239

suggested that testosterone treatments aren't likely to increase the chances of this condition or its symptoms.

Even though evidence shows testosterone treatment won't cause prostate-gland problems for most men, it's a good idea for a man to have his prostate health monitored before and during treatment with prostate exams and PSA tests. Maintaining prostate health is important—which brings us to the next topic in our exploration of men's sexual health issues. . . .

Supporting Sexuality by Preserving Prostate Health and Addressing BPH

Your partner's prostate gland is located between his penis and bladder, in front of his rectum. The largest sexual gland in his body, it can be of immense importance to his healthy, vital sexual function. When he's on the verge of ejaculation, his prostate gland secretes sperm-nourishing fluid into his urethra. At some time in his life, he may develop a normal enlargement of the prostate gland—estimated to affect up to 60 percent of men 40 and older—called *benign prostatic hyperplasia,* or BPH.

Prostate enlargement can be due to hormonal changes in a man's body as he ages, and may be caused, in part, by excess conversion of testosterone to estrogen. This conversion happens to some extent in all men, but increases with age—especially in overweight men, or those with insulin resistance (a prediabetic condition). Estrogen plays a role in the development of not only BPH but also prostate cancer. Another contributing factor to BPH is DHT, which as noted above is a by-product of testosterone. Many BPH treatments, both natural and pharmaceutical, are aimed at decreasing either estrogen or DHT in the prostate gland.

> ## Preventing Prostate Cancer
>
> Prostate cancer can be serious, but it's often curable with early detection and treatment. As you've discovered in this chapter, research shows that drinking eight ounces of pomegranate juice daily can help prevent prostate cancer, and according to the authors of *The Science of Orgasm,* higher frequency of ejaculations correlates with lower prostate-cancer risk. You've also seen that a healthy testosterone level may help prevent prostate cancer. In addition, sufficient sleep is important: a study published in the *British Journal of Cancer* in 2008 found that men who sleep under six hours a night are 34 percent more susceptible to prostate cancer than those who sleep nine or more hours nightly. The study's authors suggested that melatonin, the naturally produced sleep-promoting hormone that also has effective antioxidant and anticancer properties, may help prevent prostate cancer.
>
> A man should have a manual prostate-gland exam, as well as a PSA test, done annually beginning at age 50. (If he has a family history of prostate cancer, it's recommended that he begin these at a younger age.) A PSA test is commonly done by medical doctors on annual visits. A high reading can indicate a prostate infection known as *prostatitis,* or be a sign of cancerous cells in the prostate gland. Another test, called a *complexed PSA* (or cPSA) test, is also available, and may be more accurate.

If a man has BPH, his prostate gland may enlarge until it eventually exerts pressure on his urethra, causing an urge to urinate frequently. He may also experience reduction in intensity of urine flow and urine volume, irregular stopping and starting of urine flow, incomplete emptying of his bladder, and urine leakage after urinating.

BPH is noncancerous and typically doesn't interfere with a man's libido or ability to maintain erections, but it can disrupt his life and his sex life. He may have to urinate often in the middle of the night and be conscious of bathroom locations whenever he goes out. And the potential side effects of some prescription medications for BPH can drastically interfere with his sex life. A study published in the journal *The Prostate* in 1996 found that a commonly prescribed BPH drug, Proscar (finasteride), decreases sexual function, lowers libido, and increases impotence. And in 2004 the *New England Journal of Medicine* reported that while pharmaceutical BPH medications that decrease DHT may reduce overall prostate-cancer risk, they also render certain forms of prostate cancer more aggressive.

The undesirable consequences of conventional BPH treatments on a man's sexuality may not be limited to the side effects of drugs. In severe cases, BPH can compress the urinary canal to the point that it causes pain and requires surgery, and an outcome of surgery could be sexual dysfunction.

Considering the potentially serious effects that pharmaceutical and surgical approaches to BPH can have on a man's sexual health, it seems all the more important for your partner to maintain his prostate health and, if he has BPH, use natural remedies whenever possible. Many men with BPH experience reduced symptoms and dramatic improvement without resorting to drugs like Proscar. Let's look at the most effective natural methods of treating and preventing BPH:

— **Saw palmetto.** In mild to moderate cases of BPH, saw palmetto can be especially effective. Research shows it can help lower DHT and hinder its effects, significantly improve symptoms after two months of use, and has no side effects at appropriate doses. (At high doses, side effects may include slight nausea or intestinal discomfort.) See dosage recommendation earlier in this chapter.

— *Pygeum africanum.* An herbal medicine used for many years in Europe to treat BPH, *Pygeum africanum* contains beta-sitosterol, which has anti-inflammatory effects. Research shows it can improve urinary symptoms in many men with BPH; studies cite daily doses of 25 to 50 mg for addressing BPH issues.

— **Omega-3 fats.** As you explored previously, omega-3 fats support prostate-gland health. A man can increase his omega-3 fats with the doses of flax and fish oils recommended earlier in this chapter and by eating pumpkin seeds and walnuts.

— **Zinc.** An important supplement for prostate health, research shows that zinc can inhibit production of DHT, and help prevent BPH. The recommended dose is 25 to 50 mg daily.

— **Nettle root.** Researchers have found several mechanisms by which nettle root can help a man with an enlarged prostate gland, and reduce likelihood of BPH. The recommended dose is 300 mg daily.

Restoring Pleasure: Hidden Secrets about Circumcision and Sexual Sensation

If you assume circumcision can't have anything to do with your sex life, think again. Its rate in America—the only Western country where it's still widely perpetuated—may be directly affecting your sexual experiences with your partner. Although in some parts of the world both girls and boys undergo circumcision (the removal of portions of the genitals by cutting or surgery, usually in infancy or adolescence), in America circumcision is the removal of the male foreskin—the retractable outer part of the penis.

You might think circumcision has little to do with you personally because, as a female, if you live in the U.S., you're protected by law from all forms of cutting of your genitals without your consent—regardless of your age, your parents' religious preferences, the portion of your genitals removed, or whether the cutting takes place in medical settings. But even though you're safe from circumcision, the fact that males aren't equally protected could be impacting your sexuality in more ways than you realize.

In 2010, after nonprofit groups had fought for decades on behalf of children's rights, the *New York Times* reported the U.S. circumcision rate had plummeted to just 32.5 percent in 2009 (from 56 percent only three years earlier). This was a watershed moment; it meant that leaving baby boys intact had at last become the norm in America. Perceptions are changing rapidly, and more states are refusing Medicaid funding for circumcision, but the United States lags far behind other Western countries. For example, the estimated rate of medicalized circumcision in England is 2 percent, in Canada 9 percent, in Australia 13 percent, and in New Zealand less than 1 percent.

243

No discussion of men's sexual-health issues—and particularly how your partner's sexuality influences yours—would be complete without addressing circumcision, because even though it's in decline, males born during its peak are in their adult years. As a result, many women are still in intimate relationships with circumcised men. In the pages ahead, you'll discover how circumcision may be affecting you personally, including the immediate repercussions it may be having in your sex life, and what can be done about it.

The Sex Connection:
Why You Can't Fool Mother Nature

Like every human being, you were born with a *prepuce*—a natural part of your anatomy with important protective, sensory, and sexual functions. Also known as your *clitoral hood* (and sometimes referred to as the *female foreskin*), it covers your clitoral glans, the dome-shaped tip of your clitoris; in males, the foreskin correspondingly covers the penile glans, the similarly domed head of the penis. The male foreskin, like its female counterpart, keeps the glans that it shields soft and moist, and protects it from irritation, abrasion, trauma, cold, contaminants, and infection.

The adult male foreskin includes approximately half the skin of the penis—about 15 square inches of skin. The term *foreskin* is a misnomer; it also contains tissue *beneath* the skin that's filled with blood vessels. Let's take a closer look at the male foreskin's main functions:

— **Pleasure.** The foreskin contains thousands of delicate nerve endings that enhance sexual pleasure, including fine-touch receptors known as *Meissner's corpuscles*. According to the National Organization of Circumcision Information Resource Centers, the foreskin is the most sensitive part of the penis. It comprises some of the most specialized sensory tissue in a man's body, comparable in sensitivity to parts of your clitoris and vulva.

— **Lubrication.** The foreskin serves a unique lubricating function; it contains a type of tissue similar in structure to that of your inner lips or eyelids.

— **Mobility.** Combined with its natural lubrication, the foreskin provides a "gliding" mechanism that may aid in the entry of the penis into the vagina, and can also play a special role in sensual pleasure for both partners. Its retractable nature allows it to "roll" backward along the shaft of the penis with each thrust into the vagina, and forward again each time the penis is withdrawn. Moving against the shaft of the penis and the vaginal walls simultaneously, it serves as a kind of sensory interface between them.

— **Immunity.** The foreskin may also have immune functions. For instance, intriguing research indicates that Langerhans cells, an immune component prominent in the foreskin's lining, may help protect against infections. The foreskin appears to offer protection against infections in other ways as well; statistics suggest that you're at greater risk for HIV and other sexually transmitted infections if your partner is circumcised. (To explore the reasons behind this, see Appendix J.)

Removing the foreskin results in the loss of all its functions, and reduces the quantity of penile tissue. Without its natural protection, the glans becomes discolored, drier, keratinized (covered with a layer of "tougher" cells), and further desensitized due to continuous exposure and chafing. A study in the *British Journal of Urology* found that circumcision reduces penile sensitivity by up to 75 percent. The health risks of circumcision include infant trauma, infection (including potentially fatal antibiotic-resistant staphylococcus), hemorrhage, complications of anesthesia, and surgical mishaps that may lead to partial or complete loss of the penis, or death.

The Ethical Dilemmas

Some see circumcision as having a religious purpose—for example, as a way to designate a child as a member of a particular faith or cultural group. (The highest statistical incidence of male circumcision is in Islamic cultures.) However, routine circumcision raises serious ethical concerns because it has no proven medical benefits and deprives unconsenting minors of a natural, useful part of their bodies. Ethicists point out that the decision on whether to keep one's genitals as nature intended, along with the freedom to choose one's religion, is an individual's inalienable birthright—not his parents' or doctor's—belonging to the person himself when he reaches the age of consent. (There's only one situation in which *nonroutine* circumcision may be medically indicated for health reasons—an extremely rare condition known as *pathological phimosis,* estimated to affect fewer than one percent of adult males.)

For generations, conventional physicians claimed that routine circumcision prevents a wide variety of conditions. Science has disproven every claim, yet the belief persists that natural tissue every male is born with somehow causes health problems. All attempts to promote circumcision as a preventive measure are fraught with additional ethical problems; even if it could be proven that circumcision prevented any condition it has been claimed to prevent, it wouldn't be justified. Nowhere else in modern medicine do physicians routinely remove normal, healthy tissue from a portion of the population with the aim of preventing statistically unlikely conditions that are more effectively prevented through more conservative approaches. Circumcision, oddly out of place in a rationally based health-care system, hasn't been held to the same ethical standards and scientific scrutiny expected everywhere else.

You can learn more about circumcision, including the history of how it began in American medicine during the antisexual Victorian era (in an effort to prevent masturbation by reducing capacity for pleasure) at **www.nocirc.org** and **www.IntactAmerica.org.**

Foreskin Restoration: The Unexpected Sex Effects

If you haven't heard about foreskin restoration, you're in for a surprise. An outgrowth of the movement to end circumcision, it's one of the most fascinating consumer-driven health-care developments, full of examples of ingenuity and independent-mindedness. For a man whose right to bodily self-determination was denied by circumcision, the discovery of foreskin restoration can be a life-altering moment of self-empowerment. It can replace feelings of loss, and the sense that there's nothing he can do about his situation, with new hope and direction. It gives him the opportunity to channel his energy into a practical plan of action, and permanently restore not only his bodily tissue but also his rightful sense of self: *he* becomes the master of his own destiny when it comes to choosing his circumcision status.

Foreskin restoration is a testament to the power of positive thinking and our ability to overcome limitations—perhaps as good an example as you'll find of the inspirational attitude made famous by Louise Hay in *You Can Heal Your Life*. For some, its greatest challenge is in the mind; it takes extraordinary self-confidence to believe you can physically change the shape of part of your body. But as Louise has said, if we're willing to do the mental work "almost anything can be healed." Foreskin restoration may seem impossible, but it works.

There are surgical methods of foreskin restoration, but the term is used here to describe the more popular nonsurgical methods. These enable any man with a do-it-yourself mind-set and sufficient dedication to create a foreskin from the existing skin and tissue of his penis, using a variety of gentle stretching techniques that allow his penile skin and tissue to gradually expand and cover his glans. Men who practice restoration report increased capacity for sexual pleasure—the effects may begin to be felt within a matter of months, or even weeks. And as the glans becomes more receptive to sensation, it changes in its physical appearance: it regains its natural color and "shiny" quality as the epithelium (covering of cellular tissue) grows thinner and smoother. A man who practices restoration discovers how it feels to have his glans "internalized"—covered by the warm, protective tissue of his own body on a daily basis as nature intended. And when restoration is complete, the restored foreskin can so closely resemble a natural foreskin that it's impossible to tell the difference; after restoration, men consider themselves intact.

You can continue to explore foreskin restoration in Appendix K, where you'll find additional information about restoration methods, the science behind how and why the process works, a few important caveats, and valuable resources you and your partner can use to learn more.

When and How to Talk with
Your Partner about Circumcision

If your partner is circumcised, be especially sensitive and compassionate in your communication around the topic. Although it affects you both sexually, it's primarily *his* issue. You can work through
feelings that come up for him together, but he may understandably
have intense feelings about it, and difficulty verbalizing them. It may
make a big difference to approach the subject gently, and refrain from
asking him to discuss it before he's ready to come to terms with it.
Some men push the issue away, only to embrace it many years later.
They may eventually describe the interim as a necessary time of silent grieving for their loss. You might find that the best time to talk
about it is when he initiates the discussion; if he's confronted with the
topic prematurely, suppressed emotions may provoke anxiety, anger,
strongly expressed opinions defending circumcision, and arguments
that it should be perpetuated on other males. Or he may insist it's
not an important issue or had any effect on him, and deny he's missing anything (even though it's impossible for him to *know* what he's
missing). Another common impulse is to mask the topic with nervous
laughter and humor. It helps to keep in mind that circumcision vio-
lated his genital integrity, and that he needs your love, support, and
perhaps most of all, your empathy.

How Your Partner's Foreskin Restoration
Can Enhance Your Sex Life

If your partner chooses to practice restoration, as his penis develops new tissue and becomes more sensitive, you may notice an
increase in his sexual responsiveness and overall interest in sex.
(As one patient who practiced restoration put it, "Foreskin restoration is an aphrodisiac.") The changes he goes through can have a
direct bearing on your relationship and sexual experiences. Let's
look at the most important ways this can happen:

— **Frequency of sex.** You may find your partner desires sex
more often than he did prior to restoration.

— **Vaginal comfort.** During sex, some circumcised men require prolonged periods of thrusting to create sufficient stimulation to reach orgasm. If your partner once needed to thrust to the
point that your vagina sometimes became uncomfortably dry and

lubrication was essential to prevent abrasion, restoring the natural "mobility" of the foreskin may facilitate your vaginal comfort.

— **Condom use.** For some circumcised men, condoms further diminish penile sensation to the extent that they have difficulty enjoying sex with them. If this was your partner's experience, restoration may make him less reluctant to use condoms.

— **ED issues.** Circumcision could be a factor in many cases of ED, particularly among men in their periandropausal and andropausal years, or older. All attempts to treat ED may be limited in effectiveness if capacity for penile sensation has been dulled to begin with. According to a 2011 study in the *International Journal of Men's Health,* circumcised men have a four and a half times greater likelihood of experiencing ED than intact men. If your partner has ED, restoration may help resolve it.

— **Your overall experience of sex.** As your partner's foreskin gradually increases in size, expanding the bulk of his penile tissue, you may experience new sensations in your vagina during sex.

— **Possible psychological effects.** Restoring men often report increased self-esteem, well-being, and joyfulness in their discovery of new sensation. With time, you may notice emotional shifts in your partner that benefit your relationship on many levels.

Conclusion: Parting Thoughts on Partnership

In this chapter, you've explored many effective natural methods for enhancing your partner's sexuality with herbal aphrodisiacs and other tools. You've also explored the key sexual-health challenges he may face over the course of his life, and numerous natural solutions he can use to overcome erectile dysfunction, treat low testosterone, protect his prostate health, address BPH issues, and improve his capacity for sexual sensation.

As we suggested at the opening of this chapter, everything offered in its pages for enhancing your partner's sexuality can benefit *yours* as well. Nurturing his sexual nature nurtures your own—but setbacks to his sexual health can affect every part of your partnership. At the same time, your sexual well-being is equally important to his; the closer you grow as intimate partners, the more reciprocal your sexual energies become. A truly intimate relationship gives you the greatest possible balance of give-and-take—intimate partnership is *ultimate* partnership—and allows you to continuously co-create your sexual vitality. By upholding each other's well-being as you evolve together through the transitions in your lives, you can generate dynamic, radiant health for your shared sexuality.

CHAPTER 8

PRESERVING
YOUR PASSION
Enhancing Your Libido
for the Rest of Your Life

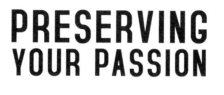

"You can have anything you want if you want it . . .
with an inner exuberance that erupts through the skin
and joins the energy that created the world."

— SHEILAH GRAHAM, *THE REST OF THE STORY*

251

Great sex, as we said at the beginning of this book, is your natural birthright; you were born of orgasm, and your body is perfectly designed to manifest sexual pleasure. This book has given you the essential tools you need to create vibrant sexual health at any time in your life, but great sex isn't your birthright on just a temporary basis. You can utilize all that you've discovered in these pages to empower your sexuality every day, for the rest of your life.

There are ways of thinking about the changes recommended in this book that will support your ability to incorporate them into your life and make them lasting and permanent. Let's look at some thoughts you can use to "frame" the contents of the previous chapters and help create change in your sexual health that never goes away.

Your Libido, Naturally:
Common Sense and Uncommon Sensuality

As your personal guide to enhancing your sex life, this book contains a lot of detailed information. But your underlying impulse to use it—perhaps what made you choose this book in the first place—is a matter of your own intuition. You may have instinctively found its natural take on sexual health more attractive than what conventional pharmaceutical methods have to offer. On a gut level, you probably resonated with its core approach to enhancing sex, which could be summed up as *natural measures, maximum pleasures.*

Far too many women let themselves be convinced that they need to use synthetic hormones or other unnatural means to regain their libido, when this simply isn't so. As you've seen throughout this book, innumerable factors and forces determine your sexual health, and you can strongly influence them with your daily choices. We've explored hundreds of safe, natural ways you can cultivate and enhance your sexual energy, from the wisdoms of contemporary natural medicine to secrets passed down to you from ancient traditions.

Your attraction to the natural approach in this book is, perhaps, also a matter of common sense and sound judgment. You may feel a basic impulse to avoid anything that runs counter to your intuitive awareness of what's natural—from drugs with toxic side effects and foods grown with pesticides, to sexual lubricants containing parabens and personal-care items laced with carcinogens.

The fact that you're reading this book shows you're on the right track, and you're making wise choices. As you move forward on your path to greater sexual health, continue to trust your common sense and follow the guiding instinct that brought you to this book. The rewards will be all-encompassing for your health and sexuality. By consistently applying the tips and techniques gathered in these chapters, you can transform your life and libido from the bottom up, at any age. Keep making the right choices during each new phase of your journey, and they'll become stitched into the fabric of your being, with never-ending benefits. This is the essence of self-help; you help yourself, and you help yourself *to a better life.*

A Call to Action: Your Rx for Great Sex

This book provides you with an enormously varied collection of steps you can take to enhance your sexuality. But you'll get the most from it, as we pointed out in the Introduction, if you use it as a whole—as opposed to referring only to certain plea-sure-nourishing nuggets of information, or homing in on specific sexual-health solutions. The effectiveness of any single choice you make to enhance your sexuality is shaped—and may ultimately be decided—by its relation to the larger backdrop of your overall well-being. One of the great secrets to enhancing your libido is that context is everything; with all things sexual, all things are contextual.

This is why some of the benefits this book offers will be most profound if you take a holistic approach, balancing and trans-forming many aspects of your health and sexuality in unison. The effects of individual aphrodisiacs you've discovered in Chap-ter 5, for example, may even exceed their reputations and your expectations—as long as you take full advantage of many of the other health-boosting and libido-liberating tools you've gleaned from other chapters. If you apply the secrets you've found in these pages from this perspective, the power of their cumulative effects may amaze you, and continue to reverberate in your life far into the future.

Of course, you won't be able to begin applying everything you've gained from this book at once, and you may want to in-tegrate some of its recommendations into your life gradually, at a pace that suits you. One of the best ways to start using it to enhance your sexuality is by choosing key elements from each chapter and making a plan—with your partner, if appropriate—to blend them into your lifestyle.

With this in mind, let's recap the main points we've addressed in Chapters 1 through 7, review the measures you can take to bring fundamental changes to fruition in your life, and reflect on how you can stay motivated to that end. This is your "call to action," if you will—an exhortation to create a strategy that will allow you to begin benefiting immediately from some of the most important options you've garnered from these chapters.

1. **Maximize your mind power.** In Part I of this book, we explored a wide range of essential tools and techniques you can use to create a stable sexual-health foundation. First and foremost, we looked at the part your mind and spirit plays in enhancing your sexuality in Chapter 1. Opening with this topic made sense; no sooner were you *opening* this book than you were *opening* your mind to the notion that your mind is capable of *opening* any door for your sexual well-being. That's a lot of "openings" for one sentence—and for your sexual health.

Your mental and spiritual well-being are vital to your sexual health; not only do they promote your capacity for great sex in a host of ways in and of themselves, but each option laid out in Chapters 1 through 7—each tool and technique you may use to enhance your health and sexuality—depends crucially on the power of your mind to choose it. Your mind's potential to make healthy choices, again and again, may be the single most influential factor in your ability to achieve great sex, and will determine the benefits you reap from every secret you've discovered in this book.

After touching on the close ties between your sexual health and your general health, and the decisive role of your psychological well-being for both, Chapter 1 delved into your mind power in more detail. Being conscious of how your brain may affect your feelings and sexuality can help you nurture a relationship—which is why we looked at key connections between your physical brain, the sway of sex-related brain chemicals surging through your body, and the intense emotions you can experience in a sexual partnership. Remember that you can harness your mind's power to build and maintain a great relationship with the means we outlined—by using time, communication, sexual trust, and support for your right brain.

In Chapter 1 you also explored your brain's *plasticity*—the physiological basis for your ability to replace negative habits of thought with new ones that promote health, love, and pleasure. As you continue moving ahead on your journey, keep making good use of this gift; with the combined effects of the methods we mapped out—allowing time for change to happen, using affirmations, meditating, and keeping a journal—you can help reshape your sexual destiny. In this chapter you looked at additional ways you can support a healthy sexual relationship by being aware of the important links between your self-esteem, behavior patterns, and sexual health. Remain mindful that you need healthy self-esteem to repeatedly make the wholesome choices that great sex hinges on—and that it's imperative to recognize the signs, and take appropriate steps, if you need to boost your self-esteem.

When you apply any of the tips, tools, or techniques in other chapters to your sex life, remember that they work best when used in harmony with everything you've discovered in Chapter 1. You stand to gain the most for your sexuality, in short, by always keeping the power of your mind in mind.

2. **Fortify your foundation.** Since every facet of your daily routines can affect your natural predisposition for sexual gratification, in Chapter 2 we explored the Great Sex Lifestyle—a way of life that solidifies your sexual-health foundation and allows you to fully bring out your pleasure potential. Without many of the features of this lifestyle, your capacity for great sex may, to one degree or another, lie dormant within you, suppressed by poor health, incessant struggles with unsexy symptoms, and compromising conditions. But by following this lifestyle on a consistent basis, you can inestimably increase the likelihood of realizing the full scope of your birthright to pleasure. Review this chapter often, and continue to assimilate its recommendations into your daily habits; the rewards can be life altering.

In Chapter 2 we profiled three key components of your Great Sex Lifestyle. First, we looked at a dietary plan that can help you manifest your potential for radiant sexual health. Continue to adhere to the Great Sex Diet—including all of its suggestions on organic food, carbohydrates, protein, healthy fats, nutritional supplements, and more—and your innate capacity for great sex will have the opportunity it deserves to shine. And remember to keep enjoying the "Dynamic Dozen" dietary choices recommended for spicing up your pro-libido diet.

Next, in Chapter 2 we looked at the sex-enhancing effects of exercise. As you put the Great Sex Lifestyle into practice, keep in mind that your body was made to move, that exercise is therapy, and that finding forms of meaningful movement can help you maintain your momentum. Balance your yin and yang exercises, and choose types of exercise, like dance, that put you in touch with your pelvis. Refer to Chapter 2's discussion of exercise whenever you need a healthy reminder of the many close connections between movement and your sexual well-being, and use it to keep you keyed up about the potential of exercise to uplift your sexual energy.

Last but definitely not least, Chapter 2 outlined another essential method you can employ to help attain the heights of sexual fulfillment you're meant to experience: with the Great Sex Detox, you can purge impurities from your home environment and streamline your body's ability to rid itself of hidden toxins that hamper your health and limit your libido. As you discovered, this can not only recharge your sexuality but also invigorate your overall well-being; by *literally* bringing out the worst in you, it can figuratively bring out the best in you. Take advantage of the step-by-step 21-day dietary cleanse that accompanies the Great Sex Detox (along with the recommended supplements and other tools) and, if you like, continue to include "magic" smoothies in your diet indefinitely.

Once you complete the dietary cleanse, as long as you maintain good eating and exercise habits, its benefits will be ongoing, and in all likelihood you'll continue to feel renewed, revitalized, healthy, and sexier than ever.

3. **Care for your core.** With your sexual-health foundation securely in place, there's a lot you can do to enhance your libido by nourishing your sexual center—the "great sex vortex" of your pelvis and sex organs. In addition to being your sexual centerpiece, containing thousands of nerve endings perfectly designed to provide you with sensual pleasure and enable you to reach orgasm, this phenomenal area of your body is pivotal in numerous other ways. It allows you to menstruate, release eggs, and procreate;

serves as your center of gravity; supports your bladder and other vital organs; and facilitates the elimination of wastes. It's also critical to your health in Chinese medicine, as the energetic nucleus of all the chi that flows through your body.

You can use Chapter 3 as a tool to help give your sexual core the attention it needs to thrive. By becoming familiar with the elegant nature of your pelvic and sexual anatomy—including your vulva, clitoris, perineum, vagina, urethral sponge, cervix, uterus, fallopian tubes, and ovaries—and understanding what you need to know to keep them in vital health, you'll be more able to bring out your inherent disposition for sexual well-being. And you're further empowered by being aware of what happens in your body during arousal and orgasm, and all the ways in which sex can benefit your health.

One of the important takeaway messages from Chapter 3 is that knowledge is power; the more you know about your feminine organs, the more you can optimize your sexual-core health and your multifaceted capacity for erotic pleasure. To this end, Chapter 3 explored your potential for multiple modes of ecstasy, and looked at the variety of ways women can have orgasms, among them the little-understood type (female ejaculation) that many women are unaware of and many doctors deny exists.

In Chapter 3 you also explored your sexual chi, and the relationship between chi and your pelvis. According to Chinese medicine, the health of your pelvis—the conduit for all the chi in your body—is of great consequence. Stay attentive to your lifestyle habits; as we discussed, you need to keep your chi abundant, stimulated, and streaming smoothly through your pelvis—and avoid "stuck chi." In addition, Chapter 3 explored how you can use simple Kegel exercises for increasing your pelvic strength and further magnifying your many-splendored propensity for pleasure.

If you encounter common pelvic or sexual-health challenges in this core area of your body—such as painful menstrual cramping, vaginal dryness, vaginitis, pelvic pain, urinary incontinence, urinary tract infections, interstitial cystitis, ovarian disorders, or cervical dysplasia—they can be notorious for causing libido limitations and sex setbacks. Overcoming these conditions can dramatically empower your health and turn your sex life around. Chapter 3 is your go-to chapter for preventing and treating them with a wide range of natural self-help solutions: herbs, nutritional supplements, dietary tips, estrogen creams, vaginal suppositories, natural hormones, Chinese medicine, acupressure, and more.

4. **Harmonize your hormones.** You can additionally boost your well-being and immensely enhance your sexuality by utilizing everything you've discovered in Chapter 4 about your extraordinary hormones—the complex, seemingly magical chemicals that are released by your glands; flow throughout your body; and exert strong effects on your biology, health, personality, sexuality, emotions, and desires. Your hormones affect your behavior and ultimately connect you with your environment by coaxing you to share your feelings, passions, and pleasures with another human being—all the while continually reshaping your experience of love, attraction, and arousal.

Creating and maintaining your hormonal harmony is one of the most important steps you can take to enhance the quality of your sexuality. As you explored in Chapter 4, your primary libido-influential hormones—the great six for great sex—are *estrogen, progesterone, DHEA, testosterone, cortisol,* and *thyroid hormone.* Remember that each plays a crucial role in your health and sexual energy, and that balance is everything. When your hormones are balanced, you tend to feel (and *be*) luxuriantly healthy, capable of achieving almost anything you set your mind to, and fully able to manifest your sexual health. If they're imbalanced, they can interfere conspicuously with your sexuality, health, and quality of life; not only are you less apt to feel sexy and vital, but some hormonal imbalances can turn potentially libido-boosting hormones into libido-busting "harm-ones."

Keeping all six of your key hormones in harmony can sextuplicate your sexual health (that is, multiply it by six); buoy your *joie de vivre;* and help you feel energized, compassionate, grounded, erotically receptive, stimulated, and empowered to use all of the other sex-enhancing secrets in this book to expand your capacity for passion.

As you go through hormonal transitions in your life, stay savvy about the many tools and techniques we've examined in Chapter 4 for nurturing and preserving your hormonal equilibrium. You've discovered that some of your hormones are more likely to be out of balance during certain phases of your life. If you experience common hormone-related imbalances—such as diminished libido, PMS, heavy menstrual flow, adrenal and thyroid issues, infertility, or midlife hormonal swings—use the methods we've outlined to evaluate your hormone levels and treat yourself with natural approaches. Be mindful that there's a lot you can do to overcome these imbalances and enhance your sexual energy, and that you may often be able to solve them with the ancient and modern measures we've explored—lifestyle and dietary techniques, nutritional support, bioidentical hormone replacement therapy, acupressure, herbal remedies, and other natural secrets—rather than by resorting to drugs or synthetic hormones.

Last, remember the inspiring viewpoint offered by traditional Chinese medicine on the hormonal changes you face over the course of your lifetime; menopause is seen as your "Second Spring," your menstrual flow is referred to as "Heavenly Water" (rather than blood), and exercise can be an effective way to dislodge "stuck chi"—which can play a part in some of the emotional symptoms associated with PMS and midlife changes (as well as the ebb and flow of your Heavenly Water). And keep in mind Chapter 4's unique outlook on how each of your critical hormones, from a Chinese medicine standpoint, can affect your body, mind, and sexuality in terms of their "energetic" yin and yang properties.

5. **Avail yourself of aphrodisiacs.** In Chapter 5, we launched Part II of this book—our exploration of numerous new dimensions you can pursue to enhance both your sexuality and your partner's. In a health-care market dominated by gargantuan pharmaceutical firms promoting products like Viagra, and with conventional doctors trained primarily to dispense drugs, there's little incentive to tell you about your natural alternatives for sexual enhancement. Yet you have a cornucopia of viable options that can transform your libido in ways no drug can. Many have stood the test of time, were cherished and carefully preserved by your ancestors, and were passed down over the span of centuries. Chapter 5 is a treasure chest of top secrets from this ancient legacy—along with some modern ones—for stoking your fires of passion to burn brighter.

Keep Chapter 5 at your fingertips if you ever feel the need for some extra sexual self-empowerment. You can always refer back to its pages, and reexplore its sex-enhancing pearls, at any phase of your life. But bear in mind that while some aphrodisiacs may boost your well-being, you'll tend to experience their greatest benefits when you're abundantly healthy. Aphrodisiacs have a way of underscoring one of this book's underlying themes—that optimal health may give you access to otherwise unattainable peaks of pleasure.

As you've seen, Chinese medicine supports this view with its notion that your level of vitality ultimately shapes your libido. (Again, take this book as a whole: try not to let the pages of Chapter 5 become dog-eared while allowing other chapters to go underexplored.) And anytime you use aphrodisiacs, remember that they're most effective when taken in the context of love, rather than simply to enhance sexuality by itself. As we said at the outset of this book, love is the most powerful aphrodisiac.

We began Chapter 5 with your "top 12" herbal aphrodisiacs from around the world—earth's generous offerings to your libido—including some renowned Chinese formulas that can revitalize both your sexual energy and your overall health. Keep in mind that some herbal aphrodisiacs directly ignite your sexuality by stimulating your genitals or increasing your nitric oxide level, while others act in less direct ways but have potent long-term results. Some Chinese aphrodisiacs, for example, may not have immediate benefits, but build your health and libido over time. And with certain Chinese aphrodisiacs, one of the great secrets is that they don't work in isolation; once again, their effects can depend on your general sexual health and well-being. To reiterate, the context of your lifestyle is everything. Whenever you seek to harness the power of aphrodisiacs, be aware of this sexual-contextual element.

Also be mindful of another secret in Chapter 5—that with many aphrodisiacs (Chinese ones in particular) the key is balance. If your sexual health is imbalanced, taking increased amounts of some aphrodisiacs doesn't always result in greater sexual energy and vitality, but can instead throw you further out of balance, exhaust your energy, and eventually reduce your libido. As a woman, you're apt to benefit most from aphrodisiacs that have a balance of yin and yang qualities, and can gradually nourish and harmonize your sexual energy.

Finally, let's refresh our memory about all the other kinds of natural aphrodisiacs and sex-enhancers we explored in Chapter 5: "gentler" herbs, flower essences, essential oils, and scents, including the hidden erotic potential of your body's own "secret" scents. We also looked at sex-stimulating nutritional supplements, foods with possible aphrodisiac effects, and "anti-aphrodisiacal" dietary items to avoid.

6. **Explore your enhancers.** To further fuel and invigorate your sexuality, you can always reexplore the many natural enhancement options you discovered in Chapter 6. Here we broadened our scope to include an array of other methods for elevating your pleasure potential—from modern to ancient approaches, from Western to Eastern measures, and from concrete, matter-of-fact means to mind-expanding practices. The tools and techniques in this chapter might not be traditionally considered aphrodisiacs, but they certainly can have aphrodisiac-like effects and exhibit many characteristics of conventional aphrodisiacs.

Many of the enhancers we explored in Chapter 6 may not only promote passion and sexual gratification, but also boost your health. Like the aphrodisiacs in Chapter 5, you can use these tools and techniques to help transform your sexual health and libido whether you currently need to recharge your sexual energy or you already have a strong libido and want to further enhance it. But remember that all sex-enhancers tend to be most effectual when your health is optimal. With Chapter 6, as with Chapter 5 (and this entire book), one of the fundamental takeaway truths is that your capacity for great health is inextricably linked with your potential for great sex. Use your enhancers wisely, in conjunction with everything you've discovered in other chapters—especially the lifestyle recommendations in Chapters 1 and 2—and their rewards may outshine all your expectations.

With its in-depth exploration of a variety of sexual lubricants—some that facilitate sex and stimulate pleasure by moistening your vaginal tissues, and others that both moisten and provide extra stimulation through more direct means—you can utilize Chapter 6 as a reference to compare products and know which ingredients to look for and which to steer clear of. Chapter 6 also gives you guidelines on using vaginal strengtheners and releasers: Ben Wa balls that date back to ancient China, where they were used to teach women exercises for fostering sexual ecstasy, and modern vaginal cones. These devices can be surprising in their ability to increase your capacity for pleasure—and multiply the effects of other kinds of sex-enhancers.

In Chapter 6 we also considered the eroticizing potential of acupressure techniques, and explored the effects of pelvic and vaginal self-massage blended with acupressure. We looked at tantric practices as well, including sexual tempo and breathing techniques that can focus your sexual energy and lift your libido to new plateaus. As we pointed out, tantric practices may not be for everyone, but if you want to explore new dimensions of sexuality and intimacy in a committed relationship, they may be right for you. According to some teachings, they can be profoundly beneficial both physically and spiritually, not only heightening your capacity for sexual sensation but also your sense of unity with the universe.

7. **Empower your partner.** In an intimate relationship, your sexuality is conjoined with his; your libidos merge, become deeply reciprocal, and you both fan the flames of your shared passions. Because you are partners in pleasure, your sexuality, in a sense, becomes mutual, and you co-create your sexual well-being. As we emphasized in Chapter 7—our penultimate exploration of your sexuality in a relationship—love and sex are all about partnership. In a healthy love relationship, you and your partner are two harmonious halves of one whole . . . each embracing, complementing, and shaping the other, your two sexual energies fitting together like the interlocking components of the yin/yang symbol. The more you know about *his* evolving sexual nature, the more you discover how compellingly it can influence your own. If his libido is healthy, it can benefit yours vastly; if his libido is out of balance, it can encumber yours in numberless ways.

With this in mind, Chapter 7 is your go-to guide for a variety of key issues that may impact your partner's sexual health. Use the tools you found in this chapter to remain vigilant about your partner's sexual-health needs, and to help both of you plot your course through the transformations he may experience over time. We examined natural methods, including herbal aphrodisiacs, nutritional supplementation, and dietary options that can empower your partner by enhancing his libido. Chapter 7 also looked at conditions that often compromise a man's sexuality, and what he can do to treat or prevent them. We focused on erectile dysfunction, explored natural treatments for it, and perused the potential consequences of drugs like Viagra on a man's health and on a relationship. We tackled the issue of low testosterone as well, including ways your partner can determine if he has the condition, its symptoms, natural means of resolving it (among them bioidentical testosterone treatment), how treatments can benefit both of you, and more.

In addition, Chapter 7 covered other important male health concerns you may need to watch for, now or in the future: andropause (male menopause), your partner's hormonal transitions, his prostate health, ways of preventing prostate cancer, and the most effective natural methods of treating and preventing BPH, or benign prostatic hyperplasia (the prostate-gland enlargement that many men over 40 experience). We also addressed circumcision, looked at its effects on sexuality (and on sexual sensation in particular), explored foreskin restoration, and considered how restoration may not only increase your partner's capacity for sexual sensitivity but affect *your* sexuality as well.

If you're in an intimate relationship, review Chapter 7 often. By keeping yourself informed of common sexual-health challenges your partner may face, and by promoting his sexual health, you can support your own sexual well-being and strengthen your relationship immeasurably.

Conclusion: Looking Back and Looking Forward

In this chapter, you've looked at thoughts you can use to "frame" the contents of this book and create permanent change. We've also issued a call to action—an overview of the primary topics illuminated in each of the previous chapters and the key steps you can take to enhance your sexual energy and vitality. This chapter has reaffirmed your ability to keep making the choices that will generate your supreme sexual health, and to apply all that you've discovered in this book to make great sex your destiny. This is an exciting challenge. When you're poised to create lasting change in your life, you're already in a transformative state—a powerful place to be. Your being is brimming and overflowing with pure potential, and anything is possible.

As you continue on your journey, you can keep using this book as your guide for recharging your libido and redesigning your sexual future. While you're moving forward, keep looking back at what you've gathered from its pages and rediscovering your power to create great sexual health. The benefits of consistently enhancing your sexuality with the secrets in this book can multiply themselves many times over, enrich your life on every level, and transcend even your wildest dreams.

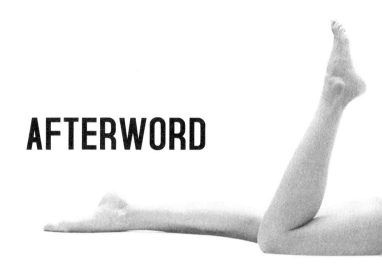

AFTERWORD

The Future of Your Sexuality:
An Upward Spiral

"When I look into the future, it's so bright it burns my eyes."

— OPRAH WINFREY, QUOTED IN CARL TUCHY PALMIERI'S
OPRAH, IN HER WORDS

Even though you have the potential to experience extreme sexual pleasure, as we underscored at the beginning of this book, there's a crucial caveat: You have to claim great sex, again and again, over the course of your life. It won't grow and blossom without your long-term commitment.

One of the central themes of this book is that your capacity for sexual pleasure and overall health are seamlessly interwoven. A healthy body frees you from countless discomforts, and gives you the energy you need to act readily on your desires—both of which are prerequisites to your ability to fully enjoy sex. As you've seen throughout these pages, great sex is a natural outgrowth of great health, and the two flourish in tandem.

Your sexuality, like your health, is part of a complex, multi-layered tapestry that extends far beyond the physical realm, encompassing everything in your life. Sex is so much more than the sum of your genital experiences; it touches your deepest emotions and desires, opens you to profound mind-body mysteries, and may connect you with your innermost spirituality. Its powerful effects reverberate in your life long after momentary erotic pleasure passes. Through intimacy, romance, and love, it can transform your behavior and feelings, reach far into your future, and forever change your destiny. This is the ultimate meaning of "great sex"— the totality of sexuality.

Great sex and great health are yours for the having; you can *choose* your way into both. All that you do—every choice you make on a daily basis about what you eat, how you exercise, and even what you think about—influences your capacity for both sexual fulfillment and abundant health. The future of your sexuality, and your health, is in your hands.

As you continue moving forward on your itinerary to more vibrant sexuality, be kind to yourself; remember that it may not be realistic to expect instant results and immediate gratification— there are no fast tracks to great sex—especially if your health is compromised and you have important challenges to overcome along the way. Keep in mind that any one piece of sexual-health advice is unlikely to suddenly propel you to peak pleasure. As you've seen, the great health that makes great sex possible doesn't happen overnight. It requires your time, patience, intention, devotion, creativity, and craftsmanship. You weave your well-being deliberately; it grows gradually, steadily, strand by strand, with each careful, meditative motion of the loom and shuttle.

At the same time, it's not a daunting challenge to claim your birthright to great sex. The resplendent health that allows you to maximize your sexuality is your natural state, and well within your grasp. This book is intended to serve as your personal "pleasure trove," by providing you with a wealth of tools and techniques for achieving the most gratifying experience of your sexuality, but the message between the lines on every page is simple: *you can create great sex and great health.*

Now that you're on your way, myriad momentum factors are working in your favor. The more you make lifestyle choices that manifest your vitality and potential for pleasure, the more likely you are to keep doing so in future situations—and to experience optimal health and radiant sensuality in any eventuality. And perpetually adding to your momentum is the fact that great health and great sex are mutually supportive, inseparably intertwined like a double helix: the higher you curve along the trajectory of one, the greater your ascendancy along the other.

Everything in this book is designed to support your momentum on this upward spiral; its pages contain the essence of what you most need to know to enhance your sexuality, now and in the future. As your journey continues onward and upward, we hope this book will open many possibilities for you and continue to expand your natural capacity for sexual fulfillment for many years. May it serve you well, and may you always enjoy all the gifts of great sex, naturally.

Aloha Nui Loa,
Laurie and Alex

APPENDIX A
Acupressure Points

Note: Some illustrations show acupressure points on one side of the body only.

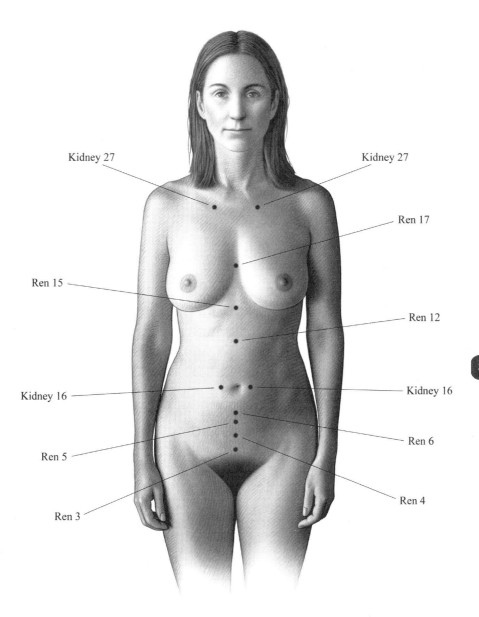

Kidney 27

Kidney 27

Ren 17

Ren 15

Ren 12

Kidney 16

Kidney 16

Ren 6

Ren 5

Ren 4

Ren 3

Acupressure points of the abdomen and chest.

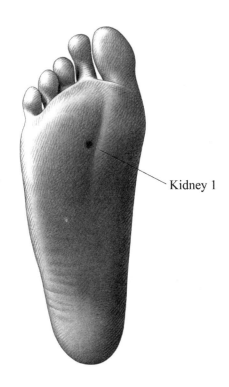

Acupressure point at the bottom of the foot.

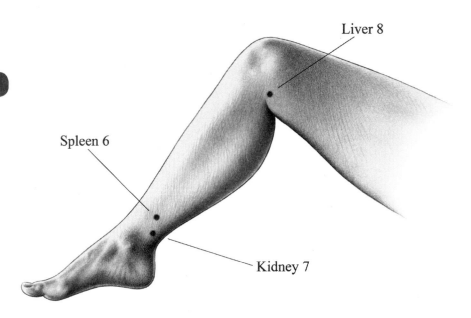

Acupressure points of the inner leg.

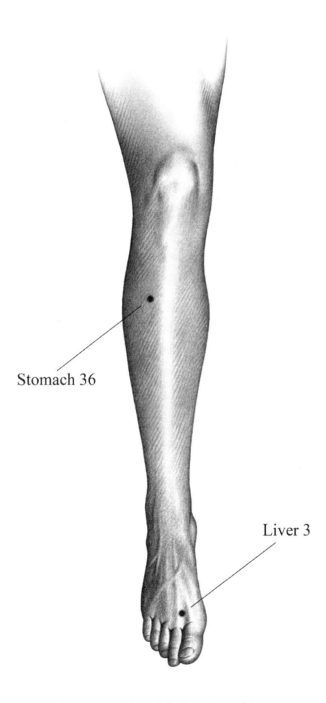

Stomach 36

Liver 3

Acupressure points of the lower leg and foot.

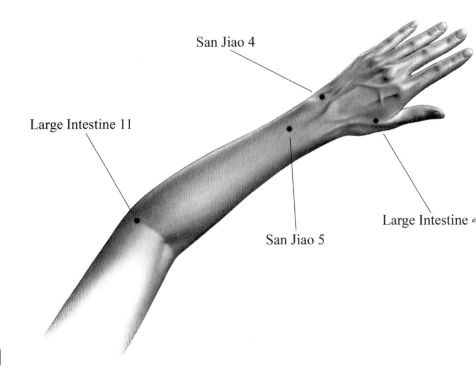

San Jiao 4

Large Intestine 11

Large Intestine

San Jiao 5

Acupressure points of the outer arm and hand.

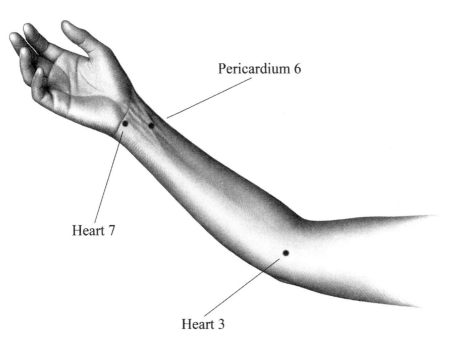

Pericardium 6

Heart 7

Heart 3

Acupressure points of the inner arm.

APPENDIX B

How Do You Find a Doctor Who's *Trained* in Natural Medicine?

Your choice of personal physician is one of your most important and potentially game-changing lifestyle decisions, but if you're looking for a doctor who offers natural medicine, you may be perplexed by your options. The popularity of natural health care has given rise to many "integrated" clinics that offer combinations of conventional pharmaceutical medicine and natural alternatives. Some may provide useful services, but unfortunately not all are what they seem.

The key question is no longer how you can find a doctor who *offers* natural therapies, but one who was actually *trained* in them. Anyone with a license to practice medicine can offer natural therapies, without ever having taken a single college course in them. Buyer beware: no government agency regulates such offers or protects you from misleading claims about natural health.

To be savvy about this, you need to understand the important distinction between licensed naturopathic physicians and conventional doctors. It's all about the education: naturopathic medical students study the same basic sciences as conventional medical students, but their education diverges sharply when it comes to the study of therapeutics—methods of treating all types of conditions—reflecting vastly different philosophies of health and disease. While conventional medical students learn to use mainly pharmaceutical drugs and surgery, their naturopathic counterparts study a wide range of natural alternatives that include nutritional science, herbal and botanical medicine, hydrotherapy, massage therapy, counseling, and other therapies.

You might think conventional medical schools have become open to alternative medicine in recent years, but research shows the curricula of most have changed surprisingly little; the focus is still on pharmaceutical treatments, with few if any requirements in alternative medicine. (If alternative courses are offered, they may be only electives.) As a result, no matter how well-intentioned conventional doctors may be, they aren't adequately trained to provide natural therapies. As Mark Hyman, M.D., concedes, "I, like almost every other doctor in the country, was trained to be a clinical pharmacologist. . . . I was trained to dispense medication."

Naturopathic schools continue to stand alone as the only medical programs requiring enormous amounts of coursework—more than 700 hours—in therapeutic nutrition and naturopathic therapeutics. Considered among the most demanding of any type of medical training in the United States, they blend rigorous study of natural therapies with much of the best that Western medical science has to offer. This makes naturo-pathic physicians—by definition, the only doctors whose *training* is truly "integrated"—uniquely qualified to offer you the full range of alternative therapies, backed by a solid foundation in the sciences.

In the United States, the only way to be sure your doctor had this kind of extensive natural-health training is to find a licensed naturopath-ic physician. It's important to verify that your doctor graduated from one of the naturopathic schools listed below, since they're accredited by the Council on Naturopathic Medical Education—the gold standard when it comes to naturopathic training, recognized by the U.S. Secretary of Education as the national accrediting agency for programs leading to the doctor of naturopathy (ND) degree. (In some states, which don't yet li-cense naturopathic physicians, anyone can claim to be a "naturopath" without legitimate training.)

— **To find a licensed naturopathic physician in your area:** Con-tact the American Association of Naturopathic Physicians (**www.natu-ropathic.org**). If you are in North America, make sure your naturopathic doctor graduated from one of these schools:

- Bastyr University, Seattle, WA (**www.bastyr.edu**)
- Boucher Institute of Naturopathic Medicine, Vancouver, BC (**www.binm.org**)
- Canadian College of Naturopathic Medicine, Toronto, ON (**www.ccnm.edu**)
- National College of Natural Medicine, Portland, OR (**www .ncnm.edu**)
- National University of Health Sciences, Chicago, IL (**www .nuhs.edu**)
- Southwest College of Naturopathic Medicine, Tempe, AZ (**www.scnm.edu**)
- University of Bridgeport College of Naturopathic Medicine, Bridgeport, CT (**www.bridgeport.edu**)

— **To find a qualified acupuncturist or practitioner of Chinese herbal medicine:** Contact the National Certification Commission for Acupuncture and Oriental Medicine (**www.nccaom.org**), or check your state's acupuncture board.

APPENDIX C
Resources

Note: Many of the products listed below, as well as some other products mentioned in this book, are available at: **www.SteelsmithVitamins.com**. Page numbers listed for *NCWH* refer to our previous book, *Natural Choices for Women's Health* (Three Rivers Press, 2005).

— **Antioxidant formula:** Steelsmith Antioxidant Formula.

— **Black-cohosh and wild-yam suppositories:** Cimicifuga-Dioscorea and Vitamin E Vaginal Suppositories by Earth's Botanical Harvest (available through natural-health-care practitioners who carry them).

— **Bone formula:** Steelsmith Bone Formula.

— **Chinese herbal wash:** Yin-care by Yao Company (**www.yincare .com**).

— **Chlorella:** BioImmersion, Inc. (**www.bioimmersion.com**), or Chlorella by Sun Chlorella (**www.sunchlorellausa.com**). Chlorella is also available from other companies at many health-food stores.

— **Eating an alkaline-forming diet:** Pages 84–87 in *NCWH*.

— **Flax and Fish Oils:** Barlean's (**www.barleans.com**) carries both flax and fish oils, and oil blends specifically for women and men.

— **Friendly bacteria (for dietary cleansing):** Theralac by the company of the same name (**www.theralac.com**; also available at some health-food stores).

— **Friendly bacteria vaginal suppositories:** Earth's Botanical Harvest Acidophilus Vaginal Suppositories by Earth's Botanical Harvest (available through natural health-care practitioners who carry them), or Gy-na-tren, over-the-counter vaginal acidophilus suppositories by Natren (**www.natrenpro.com**).

— **Herbal aphrodisiacs:** Hot Plants for Her and Hot Plants for Him by Enzymatic Therapy (**www.enzymatictherapy.com**), or Women's Libido and Male Libido by Gaia Herbs (**www.gaiaherbs.com**). These herbal aphrodisiacs are also available at some health-food stores. Libido Booster for Her and Libido Booster for Him are available through Pacific Herbs (**www.pacherbs.com**).

— **Laboratory testing:** Genova Diagnostics (**www.gdx.net**) and Meridian Valley Lab (**www.MeridianValleyLab.com**) for comprehensive hormone tests.

— **Liver lipotropic formula:** Lipotropic Complex by Integrative Therapeutics (**www.integrativeinc.com**), or Vita Lipotropic by Eclectic Institute (**www.eclecticherb.com**). Vita Lipotropic is also available at some health-food stores.

— **Making castor oil packs:** Pages 319–320 in *NCWH*.

— **Multivitamin:** Steelsmith Multi-Vitamin.

— **Other herbal products:**

- Crane Herb Company: Products by various other companies, including Two Immortals; Ba Zhen Wan ("Women's Precious Pills") under the names Women's Treasure by Jade Dragon or Eight Treasure Tea pills by Herbal Times; Free and Easy Wanderer; Antler 8 by Seven Forests; and Man's Treasure (Nan Bao Pian) by Seven Forests (**www.craneherb.com**). Products carried by Crane Herb Company are available through licensed natural-health-care practitioners.

- Dr Kang Formulas: Male Function (**www.drkang formulas.com**).

- Health Concerns: Great Yin (**www.healthconcerns.com**). Products carried by Health Concerns are sold directly to health-care practitioners, but they can also be purchased through other websites.

- JHS Natural Products: A variety of medicinal mushrooms, including reishi and a hot-water extract of cordyceps (**www.jhsnp.com**).

- Pacific Herbs: Chinese herbal products, including PMS Relief and Menopause Relief (**www.pacherbs.com**).

- Whole World Botanicals: A number of maca products (**www.wholeworldbotanicals.com**).

— **Pelvic self-massage:** *Ending Female Pain,* Isa Herrera (BookSurge Publishing, 2009).

— **Rice-based protein powder:** ClearVite by Apex Energetics (**www.apexenergetics.com**).

— **Treating UTIs naturally:** Pages 98–101 in *NCWH*.

277

— **Vaginal douche powder:** Tanafem by Intensive Nutrition (**www** .intensivenutrition.com).

— **Vitamin E vaginal suppositories:** Vitamin E Vaginal Suppositories by Earth's Botanical Harvest (available through natural-health-care practitioners who carry them).

APPENDIX D

Outline of Meals and Supplements During Your 21-Day Dietary Cleanse (for Your Great Sex Detox)

The following is a day-by-day outline of the meal and supplement portions of your three-week cleanse in Chapter 2. (Some supplements recommended can be found in Appendix C; others, as described in Chapter 2, are available at health-food stores.)

As you can see, your daily protocols change over the course of the 21 days, most notably in the number of magic smoothies you'll have daily. Depending on personal preference, you can vary your meal menus, snacks, and the way you take your flax oil, but it's essential to follow these guidelines regarding the number of magic smoothies you have each day and the particulars of your supplement routine.

— **Days 1–3.** *Breakfast:* One magic smoothie, and two lipotropic-formula pills, two chlorella pills, one capsule of antioxidant formula, two multivitamin tablets, and one antibug herbal pill.

Midmorning snack: Rice cake with almond butter.

Lunch: A large multicolored salad with skinless chicken breast or salmon, brown rice or quinoa, and a side of steamed vegetables like broccoli or kale. Add one tablespoon of flax oil to your salad dressing, or pour it over your steamed vegetables. Take at least one billion organisms of friendly bacteria, and one antibug herbal pill.

Midafternoon snack: Macadamia nuts and walnuts (a maximum of five of each).

Dinner: Vegetable bean soup with steamed vegetables, or brown rice or quinoa with fish and vegetables. Take two lipotropic formula pills, two chlorella pills, one capsule of antioxidant formula, two multivitamin tablets, and one antibug herbal pill. All of your dinners, throughout your 21-day plan, should be light, and eaten early enough that you won't be too full when you go to bed.

— **Days 4–7.** *Breakfast:* One magic smoothie, and repeat all of the supplements you took with breakfast on days 1 through 3.

Midmorning snack: An apple with almond butter.

Lunch: Salad or steamed vegetables with chicken or beans, or brown rice or lentils topped with nuts and seeds. Add one tablespoon of flax oil to your meal, and take at least one billion organisms of friendly bacteria and one antibug herbal pill.

Midafternoon snack: Coconut yogurt (dairy- and soy-free), or a handful of walnuts or sunflower seeds.

Dinner: One magic smoothie and two lipotropic-formula pills, two chlorella pills, one capsule of antioxidant formula, two multivitamin tablets, and one antibug herbal pill. If you're still hungry, have a salad or steamed greens with chicken or salmon.

— **Days 8–15.** *Breakfast:* One magic smoothie, and repeat all of the supplements you took with breakfast on days 1 through 3.

Midmorning snack: Rice cake with almond butter or avocado.

Lunch: One magic smoothie, and one tablespoon of flax oil (either in your smoothie or in capsule form), at least one billion organisms of friendly bacteria, and one antibug herbal pill. If you still feel hungry, have a small salad topped with chicken or turkey; however, it's best to have only magic smoothies for lunch, and as little solid food as possible, during days 8 through 15.

Midafternoon snack: Walnuts and seeds.

Dinner: One magic smoothie, and repeat all the supplements you took with dinner on days 4 through 7. If you're still hungry, have a small salad with chicken or salmon; but again, it's preferable to have only magic smoothies for dinner, with as little solid food as possible, during days 8 through 15.

— **Days 16–18.** For these three days, repeat the protocol you followed during days 4 through 7.

— **Days 19–21.** Repeat the protocol you followed for days 1 through 3.

APPENDIX E
Testing Your Hormones

To test your hormones, you can request that your doctor order laboratory tests. If the chart in the "Evaluating Your Hormones" section of Chapter 4 indicates that you have hormone imbalances, testing can give both you and your doctor direction on how to create optimal hormonal health. The following tests give you the most valuable information about your hormone levels:

— **Comprehensive hormone testing.** Sometimes referred to as a comprehensive hormone profile, comprehensive hormone testing is the ultimate way of assessing your levels of estrogen, progesterone, DHEA, testosterone, and cortisol. (The test measures your thyroid hormone, too, but if it shows that your thyroid-hormone level is abnormal, you'll want to follow up with the thyroid-hormone test described below.) If you're in your menstruating years, this test should be done on day 21 of your menstrual cycle to provide adequate information about your progesterone level.

The most reliable types of comprehensive hormone testing are saliva tests and 24-hour urine collection tests. These aren't generally considered "standard" hormone tests, so you may need to find a licensed naturopathic physician (see Appendix B) or other qualified holistic doctor to order them for you. Some laboratories provide saliva tests that give you information on your hormones over your entire menstrual cycle, rather than a single day only. This can be especially useful if your cycles are irregular.

Saliva and 24-hour urine tests are dependable because they measure the levels of unbound ("free") hormones in your saliva, or the levels of hormones in your urine—the best way to get a clear reading of your hormone levels. Blood tests are also available for comprehensive hormone testing, but less accurate because the hormones in your blood are bound to proteins (which means these tests don't show you how much free hormone is actually in circulation).

— **Individual-hormone saliva testing.** Any of the six hormones explored in Chapter 4 can be tested separately with an individual-hormone saliva test. If you want accurate information on your level of a particular hormone, and you don't need the comprehensive profile, this may be your best bet. As with comprehensive hormone testing, you can use this method to gauge your thyroid-hormone level, but if it shows abnormal results, you'll want to assess further with the thyroid-hormone test below.

In the case of saliva testing for cortisol, you need to repeat the test four times over the course of a day—for example, at 6 A.M., noon, 6 P.M., and midnight. One saliva test that measures cortisol, known as an Adrenal Stress Index, also measures your progesterone and DHEA.

— **Testing your estrogen metabolism.** All estrogen in your body—whether produced by your own body or taken as supplemental estrogen—is converted by your liver into either "friendly" or "unfriendly" forms. It's important to know how well you're converting estrogen: friendly forms decrease your risk of estrogen-related conditions like breast cancer, breast cysts, heavy periods, and premenstrual syndrome, but high levels of unfriendly forms are linked with increased risks of estrogen-related cancers. To assess how much estrogen you have and to measure your levels of friendly and unfriendly estrogen, I recommend a 24-hour urine collection test known as an estrogen metabolism test. This is essential if you're taking synthetic or natural hormones, and invaluable if you're a menstruating woman concerned about your hormone balance.

As you can see from the diagram below, the two predominant estrogens in your body, *estradiol* and *estrone,* can convert into one another, and into various other forms. Estrone is less friendly than estradiol because it has the potential to convert into two unfriendly hormones. The estrogen metabolism test monitors your levels of the friendly and unfriendly estrogens, as shown in this diagram.

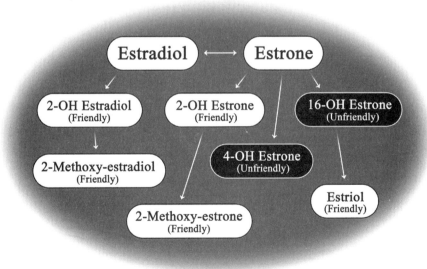

Conversion of estrogens in your body into "friendly" and "unfriendly" forms.

If your estrogen metabolism test reveals that you're converting too much estrogen into an unfriendly form, you can take many steps to support healthier estrogen metabolism. See Chapter 4 for tools and tips, including nutritional supplements and dietary changes, for promoting your friendly estrogen production.

— **Testing your thyroid hormone.** Standard laboratory blood tests can evaluate your thyroid-hormone status; in this case, blood testing is more accurate than saliva or urine testing. As Chapter 4 points out, you have more than one thyroid hormone, and your TSH (thyroid stimulating hormone) is typically tested to determine your thyroid-hormone level. If this test shows your TSH level is high, you're diagnosed with low thyroid hormone; if it shows your TSH level is low, you're diagnosed with excessive thyroid hormone.

Other tests that measure different forms of your thyroid hormone, including T4, T3 (your active thyroid hormone), and Reverse T3, can give you a more complete picture of your overall thyroid-hormone level. The most helpful tests, in addition to the TSH test, are referred to as the Free T4 test, the Free T3 test, the Reverse T3 test, and the T3 Total test. It's a good idea to have all of these done, as well as two other tests to measure your thyroid antibodies—an antimicrosomal antibody test, and an anti-thyroglobulin antibody test. The combined results of all these tests can tell you a lot about what's going on with your thyroid hormones, and the antibody tests can also detect whether you have an autoimmune condition called *Hashimoto's thyroiditis,* which can cause serious problems for your thyroid gland, resulting in low thyroid hormone.

Another tool that may be helpful in assessing your thyroid-hormone status is known as a basal body temperature test. You can easily do this test at home by taking your temperature before you get out of bed in the morning with a basal thermometer (available at many drugstores). If you're in your menstruating years, take your temperature on the second, third, and fourth mornings of your cycle; if you're menopausal, take it on ten consecutive mornings any time of month. If your basal body temperature is consistently below 97.8 degrees Fahrenheit, you may have low thyroid-gland function or a low level of thyroid hormone in circulation.

As explained in Chapter 4, if laboratory testing shows normal results but you have persistent symptoms of low thyroid hormone, a licensed naturopathic physician can offer a more thorough assessment and help clear up whether or not you have the condition known as *subclinically low thyroid hormone.*

The saliva and urine tests listed above, which may run from $100 to $350, typically aren't covered by insurance, but blood tests commonly are. For laboratories that provide hormone testing, see Appendix C.

❖ ❖ ❖

APPENDIX F
How to Use Bioidentical Hormones

As you discovered in Chapter 4, transdermal (through the skin) application of bioidentical hormones is more effective, healthier, and safer than taking them orally in pill form because it allows hormones to be absorbed immediately into your bloodstream. If you take hormones as transdermal oils or creams, they bypass your liver, circulate through your body, and go directly to your target tissue—*before* they're transported to your liver to be broken down. Thus, you need to take only the amount you actually require. Since hormones in pill form have to be taken at much higher doses in order to achieve the same effects, transdermal oils or creams result in far less hormone in your body. It's always best to use the lowest possible dose of any hormone to achieve your desired therapeutic goal.

In the case of progesterone, in addition to the transdermal oil or cream, and the oral pills known as *oral micronized progesterone* (such as Prometrium), there's a third form—a sublingual pill, sometimes referred to as a *troche,* which is absorbed under your tongue. The sublingual pill is generally preferable to the oral one, but transdermal applications are still your best bet. Every woman is unique, however, and it's sometimes wisest to stick with whatever method works for you.

An extra advantage of transdermal application is that this method allows you to have your hormones blended by a compounding pharmacy into a "cocktail" to suit your specific needs. Or they can be prepared individually, making it convenient to take them separately and adjust your dose of a given hormone at any time.

Where on your body should you apply your hormones? In the form of transdermal oils or creams, they can be applied to any thin-skinned area of your body, such as your inner arm or thigh—but even on those areas, the hormones have to pass through relatively thick dermis before being absorbed into your bloodstream. For much better absorption, you can apply them directly to the mucous membranes of your vulva or vagina; place the recommended amount on your fingertip, and gently massage it into your vulvar or vaginal tissues.

Choosing the best "base" for your transdermal hormone application is also important. Natural bioidentical hormones that you apply transdermally can be put into a variety of oil or cream bases by compounding pharmacies; when your physician orders your prescriptions, you can request certain bases. Knowing what to choose can have consequences for your health, especially if you apply hormones frequently to your delicate vulvar and vaginal tissues. Let's look at some commonly used bases, beginning with your best options:

— **Oil bases.** Two of the safest and most popular bases for transdermal hormone applications are olive oil and jojoba oil. You can conveniently apply a few drops of the mixture to your vulva or vagina each day. These bases usually contain minimal unwanted chemicals or other ingredients, and are well tolerated by most women. Other options for oil bases include grape-seed oil and emu oil (derived from the fat of the Australian emu bird).

— **NataCream.** Another good choice, this cream base—all the components of which are of vegetable origin—is free of ingredients that may be found in other products, such as solvents, chemical impurities, dioxine, and ethylene oxide. NataCream is available from Key Compounding Pharmacy in Kent, Washington.

— **PLO gel.** This cream base is frequently used for transdermal hormone applications, is readily absorbed, has a low risk of tissue irritation, and works well for many women. It contains soya lecithin, isopropyl palmitate, sorbic acid, and poloxamer 407. The first two of these ingredients are fairly benign, but the Environmental Working Group (EWG) lists the last two as moderate hazards (although they're not found in high amounts in PLO gel).

When choosing the bases for your transdermal hormone applications, you should avoid certain types commonly used by compounding pharmacies, as they contain compounds that could compromise your health. Since healthy oil and cream bases are readily available, it's easy to steer clear of those with questionable ingredients. The following bases are *not* recommended for your hormone applications:

— **Velvachol.** You should avoid Velvachol because of its high content of parabens—chemical preservatives and known environmental toxins that mimic estrogen (which means they could potentially increase your cancer risk) and can accumulate in the fatty layer of your skin. A study reported in 2004 in the *Journal of Applied Toxicology* found increased concentration of parabens in breast tumors, and subsequent research confirms that parabens are not only estrogen-mimickers but can also interfere with your hormone levels. You should also steer clear of Velvachol because it contains petrolatum, a petroleum-based ingredient; it's best to avoid using petroleum products on your body.

— **MBK fatty acid.** MBK fatty acid isn't recommended, because it contains PEG-8 distearate and hydrogenated vegetable oil. The EWG rates

PEG-8 distearate as a moderate hazard with possible links to toxicity, and hydrogenated oils are chemically synthesized trans-fatty acids that shouldn't be ingested or used on your body.

— **Vanpen.** Vanpen should be avoided because it contains the chemical butylated hydroxytoluene, also known as *BHT.* According to the EWG, BHT is a moderate hazard linked with toxicity and endocrine-system disruption; other sources indicate that it's toxic to the immune system and human skin, may have nerve toxic effects, and may contribute to the development of cancer cells. Animal studies have found that it can increase the risk of cancerous tumors.

APPENDIX G
Safe Sex, Naturally

The number of sexually transmitted infections (STIs) is greater than many people realize. In addition to HIV and herpes, they include human papilloma virus, chlamydia, hepatitis B, hepatitis C, trichomoniasis, gonorrhea, and syphilis. Some can be treated with natural techniques, others require pharmaceutical drugs, and some have no cure. Most can cause serious health consequences with wide-ranging symptoms.

STIs appear to be on the rise with the increased use of drugs like Viagra. Since Viagra became available in 1998, studies show sharply increased STI rates among the post-midlife population (the drug's most frequent users). A 2008 British study reported that the rate had more than doubled between 1996 and 2003 among people 45 or older—a significantly higher increase than in those under 45. Another study conducted in 2000 in Washington State found that the rate of gonorrhea had risen more than 18 percent among those middle-aged and older, again a higher increase than among younger people. Although these studies weren't focused specifically on Viagra, and researchers attribute the findings in part to other factors, much speculation remains about the extent to which the problem is compounded by the popularity of Viagra and similar drugs.

The safest way to avoid STIs is to be in a committed monogamous relationship—defined as one in which neither you nor your partner has any sexual activity outside the relationship. This means your exchange of bodily fluids is "private"; in a sense, you share an intimate mucous-membrane barrier that protects both of your immune systems by excluding certain aspects of the environment outside of your relationship. As long as this barrier remains in place, it's extremely unlikely that any STI will get through.

If you're in a new relationship, communication and trust are essential. You need to know as much as possible about your new partner's sexual history before having sex. But since unknowns are inherent in new relationships—even with the best efforts to communicate, you may not have ultimate certainty about your partner's sexual history—the following steps are recommended for safe sex:

— **Educate yourself.** Be aware of how HIV, herpes, and other STIs are transmitted. For example, learn what herpes outbreaks look like; you or your partner may have herpes without knowing it. Get tested for HIV, and request that your partner be tested, too.

— **Examine your bodies.** Carefully inspect yourself and your partner for cuts, blisters, sores, or other breaks in the skin anywhere on your bodies—especially in or around your mouths, hands, and genitals—which can present opportunities for STI transmission. If either of you has openings in your skin on these areas, refrain from sex until they're healed.

— **Use condoms.** Avoid lubricating the penis before putting on a condom, which can cause it to slip off during sex. Make sure condoms stay in place during sex by feeling the "ridge" at the base of the penis with your hand. Withdraw your partner's penis from your vagina soon after sex—a time that condoms are apt to come off—with one of you holding the condom's base in place.

— **Use lubrication and avoid chafing.** Lubrication prevents vaginal or penile abrasions that can lead to infections. Use water-based lubrication with latex condoms; oil-based lubrication can dissolve latex. Whether you use condoms or not, avoid anything that might cause chafing, such as excessive thrusting when your vagina feels dry.

❖ ❖ ❖

APPENDIX H
Natural vs. Synthetic Birth Control

Some people might wonder what natural sex has to do with birth control. Wouldn't it be natural to simply let nature run its course? The answer is both yes and no. Pregnancy is a natural consequence of sex without birth control, but it's also a natural impulse, exercised by people throughout the ages, to control whether pregnancy happens. Depending on your personal philosophy, you may feel preventing birth is as natural as promoting it.

If you use birth control, the method you choose can be important for your overall health. As with everything else, you want your birth-control method to compromise your well-being as little as possible. Although birth-control pills have become commonly used, they interfere with your natural hormonal balance by using synthetic hormones to prevent you from ovulating. As explored in Chapter 4, your hormonal balance is crucial to your health and sexuality. Birth-control pills also put you at risk for side effects that include irregular menstrual bleeding, depression, headaches, dizziness, breast tenderness, weight gain, and other symptoms.

There are various methods of using synthetic hormones to prevent pregnancy, but don't be fooled by the fact that they may not be referred to as "the Pill." All rely on more or less the same approach of meddling with your natural hormone levels, and can have similar symptoms. They include hormone patches like Ortho Evra, estrogen and progestin injections like Lunelle, and progestin injections like Depo-Provera.

Natural birth-control methods may seem less convenient than synthetic hormones in the short run, but they're likely to be much better for your health in the long run. And a combination of two or three natural methods can be highly effective in preventing pregnancy. Let's look at some pros and cons of common natural methods, including some that may be considered seminatural because they involve spermicide (also included are some nonnatural methods that provide alternatives to synthetic hormones):

— **Periodic abstinence.** With periodic abstinence, you simply refrain from having sex when you're most likely to conceive. You can use a basal thermometer or other methods to gauge your monthly time of peak fertility. (For more information, see *Taking Charge of Your Fertility*, by Toni Weschler.) Periodic abstinence allows for unrestricted sex any time of the

287

month except around your ovulation, but if used by itself, it's not one of the more dependable ways of preventing pregnancy.

— **Condoms.** The pros of condoms include their ability to help protect you against STIs. The cons include decreased sensation for you and your partner and possible allergic reactions to latex. Female condoms are available, although they're less effective for birth control than male condoms.

— **Cervical cap.** You can insert a cervical cap up to two hours before sex; to be effective, it has to be used with spermicide.

— **Diaphragm.** As with a cervical cap, a diaphragm can be inserted up to two hours before sex, and works effectively when combined with spermicide. If not fitted properly, diaphragms may increase your likelihood of urinary tract infections.

— **Intrauterine device (IUD).** Inserted by a physician and sometimes left in place for several years, an IUD can have the advantage of convenience. But for some women it may increase menstrual cramps, bleeding, and the risk of pelvic inflammatory disease. In some situations, IUDs may also result in perforation of the uterus.

— **Tubal ligation and vasectomy.** These methods allow for spontaneous sex without concern for birth control. If in the future you want to become pregnant, however, either method requires additional surgery, which may not be effective.

APPENDIX I

Natural Testosterone for Men: Recommended Doses, Methods of Administering, and Follow-up Testing

For most men, including men with ED or low libido due to low testosterone, the usual starting dose of natural testosterone is 50 to 75 mg daily; this can be adjusted to 100 mg daily, depending on a man's response and test results. A man should always use the smallest amount needed to achieve the desired effects. The goal is to return to his own natural testosterone level, not to oversupply his body with testosterone or produce the controversial levels some athletes seek, using testosterone-like substances, to enhance performance. (Natural testosterone treatment shouldn't be confused with the use of synthesized anabolic steroids, often taken by bodybuilders in doses many times the normal levels of testosterone.) Let's examine treatment methods for using natural testosterone:

— **Gels and creams.** The most common method in the United States, gels and creams allow a man to apply testosterone to his scrotum or anal mucosa on a daily basis. The advantages of this method are convenience of application and good transdermal (through-the-skin) absorption for most men. In addition, a man can ask his doctor to order gels or creams through many compounding pharmacies that make them. The disadvantages of gels and creams: they may cause skin irritation in some men, and you should avoid direct skin contact with areas where your partner applies them for two hours after application (since contact might affect your own testosterone level).

— **Patches.** Testosterone-releasing patches are typically applied daily to a man's scrotum, abdomen, or side. The advantages: they're relatively convenient, and available from many compounding pharmacies. The disadvantages include poor absorption in some men, visibility of the patches on the skin, and skin irritation that many men experience. Transdermal patch products that deliver natural testosterone include Androderm and TestodermTTS.

— **Pills taken orally.** Pills aren't the best way of delivering testosterone into a man's body. When testosterone is taken in pill form, most of the hormone first passes through his liver, potentially causing liver stress and damage.

❖ ❖ ❖

Two to three months after beginning any method of treatment, a man's total testosterone, free testosterone, and estrogen should be retested to make sure his testosterone level is within normal range. His symptoms should also be monitored for signs of improvement. In addition, it's recommended that he have another SHBG (sex hormone binding globulin) test, as well as a new blood test that measures dihydrotestosterone (DHT) and its breakdown products, called a *testosterone metabolites profile*. (This test, which also measures how well a man is breaking down testosterone, can be valuable in preventing potential problems associated with taking testosterone. It's available through Meridian Valley Lab; see Appendix C.)

In some cases, men who discontinue treatment find that their testosterone levels remain normal without additional treatment—in other words, they don't return to their pretreatment lows—as if temporary treatment was all they needed to jump-start their natural testosterone-producing ability. The reason for this isn't well understood, but it's worth noting that a man may not need to continue testosterone treatment indefinitely. He may want to suspend it occasionally, to see if his symptoms are resolved.

APPENDIX J

Are You at Greater Risk for HIV and Other STIs If Your Partner Is Circumcised?

As Chapter 7 indicates, statistics suggest that you're less susceptible to sexually transmitted infections, including HIV, if your partner is intact. The United States has the highest medicalized circumcision rate in the industrial world—*and* one of the highest HIV transmission rates. In Europe, where the vast majority of men are intact, the HIV infection rate is far below that of the United States. Researchers point out that the foreskin's natural lubrication and mobility reduce vaginal and penile dryness, chafing, and abrasion during sex, decreasing chances of infections for both partners. According to Intact America, circumcised men may be 50 percent more likely to infect their partners than men who are intact.

Circumcision certainly doesn't prevent the spread of HIV and other STIs; both circumcised and intact men can contract and transmit them. The proven, effective prevention methods are safe sex (see Appendix G), abstinence, and education programs about risky behaviors. Even in recent years, the media has echoed erroneous claims that circumcision prevents

HIV—a notion that may *increase* HIV risk by creating a false sense of security among circumcised men (already less apt to use condoms due to reduced penile sensation) and undermining safe-sex practices.

APPENDIX K
How Foreskin Restoration Works

Most foreskin-restoration methods involve devices worn on a man's penis, allowing its skin and tissue to be pulled downward over the glans with moderate, steady tension. Some devices, attached with tape or "tapeless" methods, use weights or elastic straps; others use "dual tension" traction devices requiring neither weights nor straps. (A cottage industry has developed to meet the growing demand, with manufacturers becoming increasingly inventive.) If a device is worn daily for a long enough time, the skin and tissue gradually stretch, eventually covering the glans.

Foreskin restoration relies on skin- and tissue-expansion principles often used by plastic surgeons. It works because gradual stretching stimulates mitosis (cell division or reproduction); the total number of cells increases, resulting in new skin and tissue. Done properly, any technique should be gentle, and not cause pain. The key is patience and long-term commitment, but the time needed varies from one man to the next. You may hear claims that some men achieve a foreskin within months, but for most it's a matter of years before they're satisfied with the results.

What often *does* happen within the first few months is that a man notices distinct changes in the sensitivity of his glans as it sheds its layer of keratinized cells—the early effects of its being consistently covered by skin and tissue, after all the years of unnatural exposure to clothing. This surge of new sensation can be powerful confirmation that he's on the right track and an encouraging preview of what's in store if he follows through with his restoration.

Foreskin restoration has centuries-old roots, but the modern movement can be traced to the early 1980s, when it began catching on in the United States. Jim Bigelow's groundbreaking 1992 book *The Joy of Uncircumcising!* sold 18,000 copies in its first printing—it can be conservatively estimated that upwards of 50,000 men have practiced restoration—and a newer edition of Bigelow's book, which remains the classic on the subject, is available.

291

Two important caveats need to be added about foreskin restoration. First, doctors aren't trained in restoration, and may discourage it, since many are pro-circumcision. (Doctors often present expectant mothers, for example, with circumcision's supposed "benefits" while failing to accurately disclose its risks and consequences.) Foreskin restoration is self-help and requires a willingness to act autonomously. Second, although it can result in a penis that looks surprisingly like it has a natural foreskin, restoration won't replace all that's lost to circumcision. The thousands of specialized nerve endings that were removed, for instance, won't grow back after restoration. (Nevertheless, some sensitivity can be regained; as Chapter 7 points out, men who practice restoration report increased capacity for sexual pleasure—as well as strongly positive emotional reactions.)

You can learn more about foreskin restoration from the National Organization of Restoring Men (**www.norm.org**).

APPENDIX L
Recommended Reading:
Great Texts for Great Sex

Cass, Vivienne. *The Elusive Orgasm*. Emeryville, CA: Marlowe & Company, 2007.

Herrera, Isa. *Ending Female Pain*. Charleston, SC: BookSurge Publishing, 2009.

Komisaruk, Barry, Carlos Beyer-Flores, and Beverly Whipple. *The Science of Orgasm*. Baltimore, MD: Johns Hopkins University Press, 2006.

Northrup, Christiane. *The Secret Pleasures of Menopause*. Carlsbad, CA: Hay House, Inc. 2008.

Steelsmith, Laurie, and Alex Steelsmith. *Natural Choices for Women's Health*. New York: Three Rivers Press, 2005.

INDEX

299

ABOUT THE AUTHORS

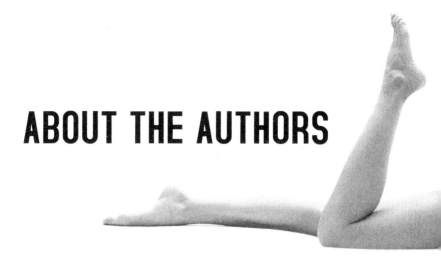

Dr. Laurie Steelsmith is a licensed naturopathic physician and acupuncturist, and coauthor of the critically acclaimed book *Natural Choices for Women's Health* (Three Rivers Press, 2005). A leading spokesperson on natural medicine, she has appeared on CNN's "Health Watch" and numerous other television and radio programs. She is frequently quoted in popular publications, including *Woman's World, Self, Natural Health, Women's Health, Whole Living, Better Nutrition, Vegetarian Times, Alternative Medicine, Health, First for Women,* and *Delicious Living,* as well as on **Oprah.com** and WebMD. She has presented hundreds of public lectures and seminars in the United States and abroad. A graduate of Bastyr University, Dr. Steelsmith has had a private practice in Honolulu since 1993. For more information, visit: **www.DrSteelsmith.com.**

Alex Steelsmith is coauthor of *Natural Choices for Women's Health* and the author or coauthor of more than 200 articles on health-related topics that have appeared in *The Honolulu Advertiser, Nature & Health* magazine, *Healthy Living Today, Vision Magazine, Hawaii Health Guide,* and many other publications. A fine artist as well as a writer, Alex illustrated *Natural Choices for Women's Health* and a number of his articles. His artwork has been exhibited in various galleries and museums, and has received many awards. You can learn more at: **www.AlexSteelsmith.com.**

We hope you enjoyed this Hay House book. If you'd like to receive our online catalog featuring additional information on Hay House books and products, or if you'd like to find out more about the Hay Foundation, please contact:

Hay House, Inc., P.O. Box 5100, Carlsbad, CA 92018-5100
(760) 431-7695 or (800) 654-5126
(760) 431-6948 (fax) or (800) 650-5115 (fax)
www.hayhouse.com® • www.hayfoundation.org

Published and distributed in Australia by:
Hay House Australia Pty. Ltd., 18/36 Ralph St., Alexandria NSW 2015 •
Phone: 612-9669-4299 • *Fax:* 612-9669-4144 • www.hayhouse.com.au

Published and distributed in the United Kingdom by:
Hay House UK, Ltd., 292B Kensal Rd., London W10 5BE • *Phone:*
44-20-8962-1230 • *Fax:* 44-20-8962-1239 • www.hayhouse.co.uk

Published and distributed in the Republic of South Africa by:
Hay House SA (Pty), Ltd., P.O. Box 990, Witkoppen 2068 •
Phone/Fax: 27-11-467-8904 • www.hayhouse.co.za

Published in India by: Hay House Publishers India,
Muskaan Complex, Plot No. 3, B-2, Vasant Kunj, New Delhi 110 070 •
Phone: 91-11-4176-1620 • *Fax:* 91-11-4176-1630 • www.hayhouse.co.in

Distributed in Canada by:
Raincoast, 9050 Shaughnessy St., Vancouver, B.C. V6P 6E5 •
Phone: (604) 323-7100 • *Fax:* (604) 323-2600 • www.raincoast.com

Take Your Soul on a Vacation

Visit www.HealYourLife.com® to regroup, recharge,
and reconnect with your own magnificence.
Featuring blogs, mind-body-spirit news, and life-changing
wisdom from Louise Hay and friends.

Visit www.HealYourLife.com today!

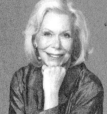
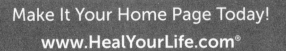